Memoirs of a Former Fatty

How one girl went from fat to fit

Gemma Dale

Second Edition February 2017

Thank you to….

my trainer Mark, who taught me what I was capable of;

Tim, for making the book better than it was before;

consultant artist Simon, for the amazing cover artwork

and Team Unicorn – the best cheerleaders a girl could ever have.

Contents

Prologue

Four years ago I was clinically obese. I was also so chronically unfit that I couldn't manage more than one flight of stairs without getting seriously out of breath and sweating profusely. I was eating my way to a whole host of health problems and my knees were knackered.

I'd been overweight since my late teens and studiously avoiding exercise since my school days.

But as 2011 turned into 2012, now in my thirties, I realised that something had to change. Four years on, I am over 80lbs lighter and a whole heck of a lot fitter. I'm now training to be a Personal Trainer so that I can help other people like me. And that is why I have written this book.

Along the way I learned a lot and came up with some ideas of my own about how and why people lose weight….or don't. I hope that you find something useful for you.

This is my story.

The Moment

Confession time. I am seriously partial to a woman's magazine. Now before you get any ideas, I am not talking about Vogue. I'm also not talking about anything even vaguely intelligent. Nothing that might include any serious interviews and subjects. I am talking about the slightly downmarket weekly type of magazine; those that usually retail for less than a pound. The type that, at least every other week, contains a story about a woman who didn't know she was pregnant and accidently gave birth to a baby down the toilet.

These magazines are simply full of people who have lost weight. There's usually an awful 'before' picture alongside a much more glamorous 'now' version. Usually, you will also find a sidebar about what the person featured used to eat before the diet and what they eat now. All this is often accompanied by some tips about how they did it. Essentially each of these stories are the same: I was really fat, I wasn't very happy, I lost weight and now life is awesome. I used to loads of eat junk food and now I eat salad and fruit. Only the photographs and the names change.

These stories nearly always have one other thing in common. Those featured have had some sort of defining moment that pushed them to change their life. For some, it was one awful photograph, perhaps tagged on Facebook for all to see. For others, it is a chair broken by their body weight. Maybe a plane seatbelt that won't fasten, a comment from one of their children, or being turned away from the rollercoaster at the fairground.

Most overweight people who go on to lose a lot of weight have generally had a moment. A moment in which something happens, something shifts and changes, and they finally decide to do something about it.

I had a few moments along the way. Several false beginnings. But there was one moment that moved me from vague mutterings and half-hearted promises (all of which had historically led to not very much at all) to actual action with tangible results.

My moment was New Year's Eve 2011. I was at a black tie dinner at my Dad's golf club. Already significantly overweight, with the Christmas Quality Street factored in I was bigger than ever. My long, black (plus size) evening dress was straining at the seams. A pair of Spanx was doing its best to keep everything in place but failing to deliver. I felt, and probably looked, like an over-stuffed sausage. My ankles were agony because of all the excess weight pushing down on them. There would be no dancing for me. Just an attempt to hide as much of my bulk as possible underneath the table and my giant wrap. During the course of the evening I went to the ladies. I sat in the cubicle and had myself a little cry. A pity party all by myself. And in that moment I decided. Something was going to change for definite this time. There would be no more false promises.

I started to make some changes. But it took me until April 2012 to get really serious. A holiday abroad in which I was uncomfortable the whole time. Uncomfortable in the plane seat, uncomfortable in the heat, uncomfortable in every item of summer clothing, uncomfortable in my own skin and with my own sense of self.

We returned from this holiday on the last Sunday in the month. I weighed myself the following Monday morning. And this is when it all began. From fat to fit. From being unable to get up the stairs without a pause in order to catch my breath to running a 10 mile race all the way. From avoiding ever looking in a mirror to finally being comfortable with who I am. From specialist clothes shops to wearing whatever I like. Being able to grab clothes off the rack with certainty that they will fit.

A journey of weight loss: a journey to a whole new self.

The Back Story

What can I tell you about me? A slightly over-indulged only child. Raised in a non-descript village in the Midlands. Genuinely awesome parents. Always loved food. All of it. As a child my nickname, courtesy of my Dad, was Mavis Cruet. If you are too young for that particular reference, it relates to a children's cartoon series called Willow the Wisp. Mavis was a rather plump fairy who loved fairy cakes. She ate so many that she was too fat to fly. I guess that tells you a lot.

A very early memory is going with my mother to the dentist for having several fillings. Followed by a conversation between my Mum and the dentist about how I needed to eat significantly fewer sweet things. A biscuit ban was discussed. A temper tantrum of epic proportions took place. The ban was never enforced.

Generally, I did well at school. I was in top set for most things apart from Maths (you can't be good at everything; that's my excuse and I am sticking to it). There were however two words that haunted my high school years: Physical Education. Otherwise known as a weekly excuse to terrify overweight or unpopular school children and reinforce the classroom hierarchy in the cruellest way possible. Not that I am still bitter or anything.

We did that thing at school when it came to team sports - you know the one, when two team captains (usually the brightest and the prettiest and the sportiest kids in the class) get to pick their team for the day, one by one. I was always, and I mean always, second to last to be chosen. Every classroom has its own structure: there is the in-crowd full of the cool kids which is followed by a strict pecking order right down the very last girl or boy. The most uncool kid, with the most uncool clothes, is dead last. Schools can be cruel places and this sort of stuff makes them even worse for those who find themselves at the bottom of the pile.

The only thing that saved me from certain last place was that I was not quite as tragic and useless at sports as the girl who was always last, who lived in the wrong street and wore the wrong clothes. Most of the time I hung around with the cooler crowd of kids, from which someone would eventually take pity on me and put me in the least damaging position in the team.

When it comes to sports I have one big problem; a total lack of hand-eye co-ordination. If you throw a ball in my direction you can be fairly sure it will bounce straight off the side of my head. If I throw one to you, it might go straight to you or equally it might be fifteen feet to the left and I can't see any difference between the two. This pretty much ruled me out of everything we did at school from rounders to netball to tennis to badminton. My standard position in netball was Goal Defence. Which basically meant I was as far away from both goal and ball as possible whilst still actually being on the court.

The only thing that my terrible co-ordination skills didn't rule me out of was swimming. Only I'm also claustrophobic. The idea of putting my head underwater, where there is none of that oh-so-important oxygen stuff, fills me with horror. This didn't present much in the way of trouble when we first took swimming lessons at school, when all we were required to do was go up and down, side to side. But then came that rite of passage required for all teenage school children. The requirement to go to the swimming baths in your pyjamas and dive for a brick. I never achieved it. To date I don't appear to have missed out as a result of failing this vital part of my education. There have been precisely no times at all since I was 14 and finally shamed from the pool, that I have walked past a swimming pool in my nightwear and spotted an urgent need to save a drowning piece of masonry.

Of course you had to pass the brick test before you could do any more of the swimming activities. For a whole year I had to swim by myself in the shallow end whilst my classmates went on to bigger and better things. In the end, the humiliation got too much, and my mother wrote me a note saying I had my period. Every Monday afternoon for a year. The school was on the verge of sending me to a gynaecologist when term ended.

My other utter embarrassment was badminton. The hand-eye co-ordination thing impacted there too. I would drop the shuttlecock and swing the racket, but never the twain would meet. I once even hit myself in the face with the racket. In the end when everyone else progressed to playing doubles matches, I was made to stand in the corner hitting the shuttlecock against the wall. When I could make it connect with the racket that was (the shuttlecock, not the wall. Even I couldn't miss the actual wall. Probably).

Instead of trying to overcome any of these issues, it was easier to hide from them. I made excuses to get out of the class. I goofed around and took the mickey out of myself before anyone else could. I pretended that I didn't care. I became adept at tactics to get out of anything physical. Once we had cross country running around a park near the school. I ducked off through a pathway between the houses, walked home and got my mom to drive me back around to the school gate half an hour later. When we did field sports in the summer and we were supposed to run laps, instead of even trying I just deliberately walked it as slowly as possible, coming in last whilst everyone else lay on the grass waiting and the teacher fumed.

The PE teacher was vile. She actively despised me and my attempts to get out of her activities. She was not averse to commenting on my abilities (or lack thereof) in front of the whole class. I sometimes wonder what might have happened if she had reached out to me instead and tried to show me a better way or helped me overcome my fears.

But the die was set. This was my approach to anything resembling exercise for years. It wasn't me, it wasn't part of my plan. It wasn't until I came back to exercise again in my mid-thirties that I realised that there was a lot more to it than team sports, unruly balls and embarrassment.

So in summary, school sucked big time. Some people say they are the best years of your life. They definitely weren't mine. They were times of wishing to be somewhere, anywhere else.

Putting it on

My Personal Trainer weighs me every Monday morning. After a particularly indulgent weekend which had led to a fairly epic weight gain in just seven days, he looked at me and asked: '*What did you eat?*' And I thought to myself that this was a very stupid question. Because the answer was simple: *all of it*.

People gain weight for all sorts of reasons. There's no simple answer as to why it happens and everyone is different. For me, I ate too much because I liked it. There was nothing more complicated about it than that. I liked it and I wanted it so I ate it. And despite all the life style changes I have made over the last few years, sometimes I still do.

It might seem strange thing to say but I'm not sure I realised just how big I really was for a very long time. I was firmly in denial, busy telling myself lies. My weight crept on so slowly that it was barely noticeable, to me at least.

I went off at eighteen to university, as you do. And it was there that my weight first began to get seriously out of hand.

Too many late night pizzas. Too many pints of lager. Not enough (or really, any) exercise apart from a Friday night bop in the student union. This was the start of years of being unable to buy nice clothes. Or eventually many clothes at all. Years of opening the wardrobe, trying things on and then tossing them on the floor, wanting to cry. Years of silently accepting the next size up. Of being everyone's fat mate. Of making the self-depreciating jokes before anyone else had the chance to.

Like most students I spent my three years at university largely focused on having a good time. Only the occasional annoyance of having to attend a lecture or write an essay got in the way. At the end of the course I left after acquiring a degree in law without any intention to follow a career in it; the ability to walk in a straight line after five pints or lager and an additional two stones in weight. As I had absolutely nothing better to do I became a recruitment consultant. A job that involved very little recruitment and even less consulting. It did however involve a great deal of sitting at a desk and making sales calls. To contribute further to my weighty downfall, the office was also next to a Greggs. Mid-morning pasty anyone?

During those first months at work my weight did go down a little in spite of the regular trips for a cheeky sausage roll. It wasn't especially because of anything that I did, it was just driven by some natural changes of lifestyle, namely less lager and fewer lazy lie-ins. It didn't last. Up and up my weight crept, starting to get seriously out of hand in around 2005. Size 16, then 18, then 20…. and then there is nowhere left to go but those stores for larger ladies and specialist bra shops that sell only giant boulder holders.

Up and up went my weight.

The Impact

An increase in size naturally leads to a decrease in energy. I got up, went to work, sat at a desk, came home, put my pyjamas on and sat down some more until it was time to go to bed. Which was about nine o clock most nights. I was constantly tired.

I entered into a long term, co-dependant relationship with my sofa.

If I went out, I went out to eat. I was always up for restaurant food. But slowly all of the other things that I loved just dropped away. The loud, fun, happy girl that I used to be disappeared somewhere along the way and was replaced with someone who was lonely, sad and anxious.

My drug of choice would vary. I had a tendency to eat one particular very bad food and over-indulge in it for weeks before casting it aside for something new. In no particular order my own sweet and savoury downfalls included Boost bars, Matchmakers (mint: never, ever orange ones) large chocolate Buttons (family size bag, obvs), Ben and Jerry's Caramel Chew Chew, Mars Bars, sausage rolls (Greggs) and lemon bon-bons. I once ate so many of those that I didn't go to the toilet for three weeks. My insides consisted almost entirely of toffee. The Ben and Jerry's obsession lasted the longest. A tub a night. At those prices, I am surprised that we could afford the mortgage.

Naturally, there were consequences of my weight gain. The first of them was gallstones. Anyone who has suffered with gallstones knows that they are excruciatingly painful. Lots of people call an ambulance during their first attack because they actually think they are dying. Mine appeared when I was about two years into my weight loss journey. I didn't know at the time but is actually quite common for people who have been overweight and then lost it to suffer from gallstones. It's a particular complaint following weight loss surgery when weight is lost very quickly. Surgery to remove my gallbladder put me back a little. Somewhat naively I had convinced myself that an operation as a day patient by keyhole surgery couldn't be that big a deal. How wrong I was. It took me weeks to feel normal again, as well as feeling like exercise. The first time I went swimming after the operation I turned onto my back to do back stroke and promptly sank as I no longer had the stomach muscles to hold up the weight of my head and shoulders.

My weight had also given me dodgy knees. They were quite literally buckling under my weight. As a further part of the whole denial thing that I was firmly invested in, I didn't realise it was because they were carrying around so much bulk. I thought instead I was developing arthritis. Funny? Perhaps if it wasn't so ridiculous.

There are lots of things that being overweight takes from you. Some big and some small. Being able to wear high heels. Taking pleasure in shopping for clothes. Being able to wear anything remotely fashionable. Being able to buy a bra in a normal shop. Being able to walk up a flight of stairs without stopping to catch your breath and the back of your neck getting damp with sweat.

These changes happen so slowly that you barely notice them happening. You tread a slow path towards obesity and sadness, barely even noticing each sad little step.

By 2012 I was in a size 22. I could only shop in specialist clothes stores. My bras could house a small child, my jeans comfortably double as a tent. I couldn't easily climb a flight of stairs.

And I was very, very sad.

I tried diets. Or I pretended to at least. I was partial to a dramatic announcement that I was, *sound all of the klaxons,* 'GOING TO LOSE SOME WEIGHT'.

I joined Weight Watchers once. I went to my first meeting held in a local school hall near my office. Paid the money, had my initial weigh-in, got the books and the special points calculator and listened to the motivational speech. I joined in with applauding those who had lost weight since the previous meeting. It all sounded excellent. I'm not sure I was entirely committed to the process though. One of the colleagues that I went with is fond of reminding me that on the way out of the meeting I telephoned my other half and told him to put a steak pie in the oven. I hadn't even made it out of the building before I was cheating. I persevered with their points system for a while but it didn't work for me. My main problem was that the book gave you the points value for all the really bad food too. So I very quickly figured out the points value of everything from a Mars Bar to a McChicken sandwich. And I ate them rather than lettuce. I'd usually have eaten my entire permitted food amount by say, 11am. It was my one and only trip to the school hall.

Then there was the juice detox diet. This was sure to work. After all, didn't all the celebrities do it? So I ordered three days' worth of juices all to be delivered frozen. I figured that even I could stick to three days of just drinking juice. They arrived. Juices based on broccoli and spinach. Others based on carrot and beetroot. And every single one tasting like the devil himself had invented a drink for the sole purposes of torturing the souls of the unworthy. Imagine drinking thick, gloopy, cold carrots. I drank each one with a bin by the side of me to throw up in, so sure was I that my digestive system would never tolerate such foulness. By day two, the vegetables were fermenting in my stomach. Certain lower bodily emissions were a regular occurrence. My belly was so swollen I looked like I had a beach ball up my frock. On day three I decided I would rather be fat forever than drink one more bottle of frozen green sludge. The rest of the bottles went in the bin. Which is where I might as well have put my £120.

Then there was the 5:2 diet. With the enticing promise that if you could just restrain your inner piggy for a 24-hour period twice a week you could eat what you liked the rest of the time. The unintended consequences of that diet were a vile headache and even more vile temper. The day following a fasting day I felt sick and faint all day. I'd lose a pound or so, but then put it straight back on once I returned to more typical eating. I tried for a week or two but I gave it up before my other half moved out.

I also tried drinks that were intended to fill you up in order to help you eat less. They came in sachet form and cost me the best part of £25. You mixed the powder with water and then drank it – three times a day. In terms of taste I'd liken them to cleaning the toilet bowl with your tongue (I assume, for clarity I have never actually done this). One day I made a sachet at work but before I had the chance to drink it had to go to a meeting, leaving it on my desk to ferment. An hour later I came back to find it had expanded right out the plastic cup, and was now a fluorescent pink thick ectoplasm. Think Ghostbusters and you will know exactly what I mean.

These weren't the only diets and quick fix solutions I have tried over the years. I know that some of these diets have worked very well for people, and they have found them of much greater benefit than I did. But here's the thing. Every single time I had tried one of these diets, I hadn't changed my underlying beliefs or behaviours. I wasn't committed to making lasting change. Hell, with the Weight Watchers attempt the hoped-for behavioural change didn't even last as far as the car park. If you change how you think about food and exercise, then you can lose weight and achieve your dreams. If not, you will just be going through the motions. I can remember talking about going on a diet and following it up with an additional comment along the lines of 'only it never works and I never stick to it'.

So I got exactly what I subconsciously expected and believed.

Nothing.

The second worst day in the world, ever.

I reflected earlier that many people have some sort of trigger that makes them lose weight or decide to take another path in their life. But there are often other moments along the way. Sad ones, miserable ones, ones that you would like to forget. Moments that should perhaps have led to change but didn't.

One of the worst experiences of my life should have been one of the best; choosing my wedding dress. Something that little girls dream about. Only mine was more of a nightmare than a fairy-tale.

Any bigger girl who has got married will know that wedding dress shops usually stock one each of the dresses they sell. Typically these dresses will be a size 10 or a 12. Maybe a 14 if you are lucky. But not all that much in an 18 or above unless you can find a specialist shop. In recent years I've seen more for the larger bride but there wasn't much about at the time when I was shopping.

My mum and I went out for what I expected was going to be a wonderful day. I quickly realised in that it was going to be anything but. There was simply nothing for me to try on. We went from bridal shop to bridal shop. The assistants were for the most part kind. But honest too. They just didn't stock my size.

A horrible sinking feeling settled in the pit of my stomach. Tears close to the surface.

Rummaging in one shop we found a size fourteen. It wasn't a dress but a two piece skirt and corset. The corset undid all the way down the back. Picture this. I am in the fitting rooms, wearing a voluminous skirt that is at least two sizes too small and doesn't do up. The assistant whips off my bra, and holds the corset around me. It also doesn't do up. It isn't even close. In fact there are about six inches of flesh between one edge and the other. All the same, she shuffles me out of the fitting room into a packed shop to show my mother what I look like. There I stand, big knickers on display at the rear where the skirt doesn't fasten. Bare skin on display at the back and massive bosoms nearly falling out the front. She might as well have shouted 'look at the fat girl who can't get the dress done up'. Everyone in the shop stared at me. Or maybe they didn't and it just felt that way.

The dress was horrible. It was nothing like the one that I had always wanted; the dress I had dreamed of when playing at being a bride as a little girl, with a piece of net curtain for a veil. It had big shiny swags down the side like a pair of tragic curtains left over from the 1980s. I bought it all the same. I just wanted to get out of there and forget this day had ever happened.   And I did not want to try anything else on, even if there had been another option - which there wasn't. Hanging half way out of a wedding dress was as close as I got to trying on beautiful lace gowns until the one I had ordered had arrived. Only by then I'd put even more weight on and it was too small and had to be sent back for a bigger version. Most women lose weight on the run up to their wedding. I am the only person I know that got fatter instead.

Even the horror of that day didn't prompt me to do anything about my increasing size. The wedding itself was a lovely day. But my feet ached badly as I was really too heavy for the pretty heels I had bought to go with the dress. The beading on the bodice dug into my bingo wings, leaving sore, scratched patches all down my arms. As all weddings do, the day involved a great deal of posing for photographs, a process despised by many overweight people, me included.   Double chins everywhere.

There are no wedding pictures on display at my house.

The day that was even worse than that one.

One of my colleagues asked me to step in for her at the last minute and attend a customer function. My employer at the time had sponsored an award at said customer's internal employee awards and I was to be the person who presented it.

When you are big you don't really like people looking at you all that much. You like standing on a stage in front of a room full of people and having your picture taken even less. The last minute nature of it meant there was no time for emergency dress shopping. Something out of the wardrobe would have to do. Along with my trusty Spanx (two pairs of). Ever conscious of my stomach, I took with me a large wrap and was sure to wear it draped loosely around my stomach area. Along with some strategic handbag holding I thought I had done a reasonable job of covering up the worst of my squishy bits in the photograph.

After I had done my corporate duty I decided that a well-earned cigarette was overdue. Standing outside the front of the hotel and lighting up, one of the other party goers started to chat to me. And then she uttered the words. The words.

"When are you due?"

Yes.

I was so fat she thought I was pregnant.

When I told her I wasn't expecting I was just fat she was embarrassed. But probably not as embarrassed as I was. I swore I would never tell anyone that happened. And yes. I went home and cried. I'd actually lost some weight by this point, probably a stone or so down from my heaviest weight. And I swore that no one would ever ask me that question again.

False Dawns

From time to time during my bigger years I would begin - with good intentions and much vigour - an exercise regime or healthy eating plan.

There was the exercise bike that I purchased, thinking that I could cycle away in the comfort of my own home whilst watching the television. Installed in the corner of my bedroom, instead it became a handy clothes hanger. So much quicker than putting things in the wardrobe!

Then there was the actual bike that I asked for as a birthday present whilst at university. It went for a little trip around the village and then it went into the shed. Where it stayed until the tyres rotted right through.

Next came the abdominal crunch contraption. That gathered dust for a while in the spare room. Then it went to the charity shop waiting room (a.k.a. the loft). Until it eventually made its way to the actual charity shop.

Along the way, as well as false starts there were also a few rock bottoms. Incidents, some small and some not, that should have encouraged me to get off the sofa. You sometimes think that you have hit rock bottom, like being mistaken for someone six months pregnant, but then you realise there is another level even further beneath that after all.

There is one big (literally) problem when it comes to weight loss. It takes a long time to achieve it and to see it within yourself. Sustainable changes are not immediate. Chocolate on the other hand is. This disconnect is part of the issue. Eating the chocolate is a form of self-sabotage. Each and every mouthful, or each and every treat, is taking you further and further away from what you really want. You have to choose what you want most. The immediate fix, or the long term result. All too often, we lose sight of the long term goal when the quick and easy thing is just asking to be eaten right now.

Usually this it is all about readiness. There are stages to change. If you do a quick Google search there's plenty written about it. One of the simplest is the 'Readiness to Change Model'. Without boring you with too much theory, it basically says that change starts with simply thinking about making a change: the initial interest or a particular trigger. The individual might then do a little preparation. Buying some new trainers for example. Downloading a fitness app. Checking out the local gyms or weight loss classes. The next stage of change is actually doing something about it. But this is where a lot of people get stuck. They make one or two changes and then come up against a barrier or see no difference and give up. Perhaps because they are not truly ready to make the change.

Those that do well, that go on to lose the weight or run that half marathon, stick with it and make it a habit. They find themselves in the hypothetical success pages of the weight loss magazines. They maintain the change, and if they fall off the wagon they get right back up and on it again.

More about habits later.

Finally, doing something about it.

I've told you about the main moment. The final (cheese) straw that broke the camel's back. And then it all began. To quote a song, I decided to burn an effigy of everything I used to be.

Throughout this little book, I've talked of losing weight and getting fit as being on a journey. I'd like to apologise for that as it's all a little bit X Factor. But it does feel that way. An ongoing, lifelong journey of change.

As I've already said, even though I had my moment of truth on New Year's Eve I didn't take any serious steps until April that year. A holiday abroad in which my weight left me overly hot and bothered and finally pushed me from contemplation to action.

I stood on the scales on return from that holiday, noted my weight and began. I did not start a diet. I did not follow a plan or join a group. I simply downloaded My Fitness Pal and started to log what I ate, beginning with figuring out how many calories I was actually consuming every single day (on an average week day an easy 2500, on a weekend, much, much more).

Slowly, slowly, I reduced my calorie intake. I ate according to my goals and removed one bad habit at a time.

Disclaimer time. If you have purchased this little book hoping for a miracle cure or some secret that no one else knows about how to lose weight and keep it off, then I guess it's time for me to confess. Because I don't have one*. Because there isn't one. You just to have make enough changes and better choices.

All. The. Time.

We use the word 'diet' wrongly. The dictionary definition of diet simply means what we eat. But we use the word instead to describe a specific eating plan. An approach. Something that is for a defined period of time. Something with an end point. One of those things that we begin (and often end too) in January after the Christmas over-indulgence. And that is where we go wrong. Because if you want to lose weight and keep it off, it is about making changes that you can live with, for life.

I ate less and I moved more.

And then instead of eating simply less, I ate well. Then I moved even more.

Slowly, slowly, the number on the scales reduced.

A pound or so a week, most of the time.

Every stone represented a new victory. Every reduction in dress size was a personal triumph.

One habit at a time.

Small steps.

Keeping on going.

I'm writing this particular chapter in March 2016. Which means that next month, it has been four years since my journey properly began. You might be reading this thinking that is a very long time. And it is. During these months and years I have lost to date six stones. In the early days it came off fast. In the last year or so it has been much slower. Those final four pounds that will get me to my target weight are still eluding me. I'll get them, sometime or other.

I have gone from a dress size twenty two down to a size ten. Most of the time. Once, even a size eight, although that particular excitement has yet to be repeated.

Goodness only knows what I have lost in terms of inches and body fat. It's something I now wish I had recorded when I first started to make changes in my life.

But here's the thing: when it comes to losing weight, it isn't just about losing pounds and inches. It is also about dealing with the reasons that you put it on in the first place, and why it has stayed on. And that is a whole other ball game.

*Sorry about that. You could try asking Amazon for a refund.

Magical Moments

The first time someone asks *"have you lost weight*?"

Wearing a dress for the first time in years and feeling okay about it.

Losing that first 10lbs.

Going under another stone, another dress size.

Taking clothes that are too big for you to the charity shop.

Looking at old photos and realising how far you have come.

The first time someone asks you for advice.

Realising that you are no longer out of breath when you run up the stairs.

Zipping up your very first pair of knee high boots.

Realising that the strange sensation around your waist whilst running on the treadmill, is your jogging trousers falling down.

The first holiday where you don't have to cover up on the beach.

The first competitive race, standing on the starting line with hundreds of other people and realising that you belong there too.

Catching sight of a girl in the mirror at the gym, squatting with a bar across her back and realising that it's you.

Knowing that against all the obstacles, you did it.

Relapse

If you have read the few last chapters then maybe you'd be forgiven for thinking that the last few years have all been plain sailing. That I have got this stuff all figured out.

Well that ain't necessarily true. I just prefer to remember the good bits of the journey.

I have relapsed several times. I expect to do it again in the future.

Let me tell you about Christmas 2014.

Like many workplaces, at Christmas we have one of those days where everyone brings a little bit of something to eat. Where I come from it's called a Fuddle. So when it got to our team Fuddle in mid-December the office was full of tempting treats. Quality Street by the tub full. Sausage rolls, crisps, cheese, dips, cakes, biscuits. Lots of bread. And oh, so much chocolate.

We didn't even wait until lunch time. About 11am we laid out the spread and I began to eat. And I didn't stop until the 2nd January.

I ate *everything*. I worked out later that on one day I consumed 1500 calories through strawberry and orange Quality Street chocolates alone. Mince pies, Christmas cake, cheese footballs, pigs in blankets, puddings and custard, crisps, nuts, marzipan fruits. I don't even *like* marzipan fruits. The house was filled with all of those foods that you wouldn't buy at any other time of year. And I ate it all. If something didn't move for more than five minutes I stuck a fork in it and scoffed it. Then there were the Christmas nights out and all of the seasonal booze. I worked out in the gym every day apart from Christmas Day itself. But no workout could off-set the sheer volume of calories that I was consuming.

Christmas came and went. New Year's Eve too. The cupboards were finally bare. And then there was nothing left to do but get on the weighing scales and face it.

Ten pounds. 10 whole pounds. In less than three weeks.

Ten pounds that had taken me months to lose in the first place.

Weight and guilt: a toxic combination.

So much guilt.

Wondering why you had eaten it.

How you had gotten quite so far out of control so fast.

Why you had undone all of your good work.

Reverted back to all your old habits.

How easy it had been. How enjoyable it had been.

The temptation to just give up and give in: so strong.

To eat even more.

I had eaten all of those things that I loved and missed. That I deprived myself of every single day.

But I didn't give up. I started again. It took me a couple of weeks to get half of that weight gain it off. Much longer to get rid of the rest of it.

And do you know what? I did it all over again the following year.

There are some lessons that you learn, there are some mistakes that you are destined to repeat.

My thoughts on relapse are these:

Shit happens.

It isn't the relapse that defines you, it is whether you give up the fight or carry on.

So put your big girl or boy pants on and deal with it.

Put it right.

Because at least this time you already know that you can.

Crap that people have said to me as I have lost weight.

During the last three and a half years, lots of people have had something to say about what I have done. Some of it was supportive, constructive and useful. Some of it was distinctly less so. Most of the time I smile and say something nice back. Sometimes, I am a bit ruder.

Here are some of my favourites along with what I say in response, even if sometimes it's only in my head.

I feel really sorry for your partner, because of how much time you spend in the gym.

Well, the last time I checked he was making the most of having the remote control to himself.

I'm your fat friend now!

Yes. You are.

When are you going to stop?

Stop what? Stop getting healthier, reducing my chances of getting life threatening illness, improving my strength and resilience, feeling great about myself? Not any time soon, but thank you for asking.

It doesn't suit your face.

Erm, thanks for that.

You are going to get anorexia.

I'm probably not actually. Anorexia is a serious mental health condition. I don't have it.

You are disappearing. There is nothing of you.

Looks in mirror. Yep, I'm still here!

I bet because you work out, you can eat as much as you like.

Yes, it works just like that. Not. At. All.

What I find interesting is how it is seen as somehow acceptable to make these sort of comments to people as they are losing weight or already thin. Things we wouldn't say when people are big or getting bigger. Either way it is a form of body shaming and says more about the speaker than the recipient.

Just a thought.

The Shift

When I began this journey, it was all about being thin. That was the end game. It was about wearing nice clothes again. About not sweating and getting out of breath all the time. About not hiding from a camera. Being thin was my answer to everything, or so it seemed at the beginning.

Somewhere along the way, in the middle of 2014 something shifted. I'd lost about four and a half stone by this point. And this is when it stopped being just about the number on the scales and started being about how strong I was; how strong I could possibly be. It was about being toned. About what my body might just be capable of.

During what I now think of as the 'sofa years' I never thought about exercise. I was still stuck in that old mind-set. I was still that girl at school, trying to get out of PE.

Despite my legendary reluctance to doing all things physical, I'd been a regular in the gym for a while by this point but wasn't entirely sure where I was going with it all. I'd done a Race for Life 5K too, in the summer of 2014. That was an interesting experience. I'd never even run for a bus previously.

Of course I got around the course, in a reasonably respectable (for me) just-short-of-45 minutes. I managed to run a reasonable amount of the course and only felt like dying for about half of it. I hadn't had a time in mind. It hadn't occurred to me until the morning of the race. I had a text from my Dad as I drove to the event. He told me he would double my sponsorship money if I came in sub 45 minutes. I laughed it off but immediately resolved to do it all the same. As I came towards the end of the course, tired and hot and with sore feet, I looked up and saw a big digital 43.45 across the finish line. I summoned up the last bit of energy that I had and sprinted the last 100 yards. And I enjoyed every moment of asking for that extra sponsorship money.

This is where it started; where my story becomes more about fitness than weight loss alone.

To Sainsbury's and back

I first began to run in preparation for the Race for Life. I knew nothing about running. I just put some trainers on a started to move and hoped I didn't look too much like an escaped hippopotamus.

Not too far away from my house is a small Sainsbury's. I decided to see if I could run all the way there and back, a combined distance of less than a mile.

Running there wasn't all that awful, mainly because it's pretty much downhill all the way. Running back again (or more accurately, shuffling back) wasn't quite so good. I had to stop four times to rest and breathe. Arriving home red, sweaty, exhausted and having taken an age.

The shop sign was my focus. Big and orange. All I had to do was get there and then all I had to do was turn around and do it again. Easier said than done.

That became my goal; to be able to run all the way to Sainsbury's and back without stopping. It took me about a month of running it two or three times a week before I could do it.

On the day of day of the Race for Life itself I didn't know where to go without something orange in the distance to aim for.

Now as I prepare for my half marathon, the distance seems almost laughable. What a big deal I made of it, running just to Sainsbury's and back again. But that's the thing about running. You get better and you get faster and then you don't want to stop.

It was only to Sainsbury's and back. And the start of a whole new part of my life.

Running and Me.

A few months after the Race for Life 5K, I joined the beginners group with Sweatshop. They offer a nine week course with the aim of getting you to run a 5K non-stop. The training is interval based. Run some and walk some, with the running element increasing week on week. At the end you graduate into the 5K running group, and get your Sweatshop running community t-shirt. A t-shirt that proclaims you to be the member of a running community. Me. The girl who couldn't get picked for the netball team. A member of the running club. I'll take that, thank you.

The people I'd joined with didn't keep it up for long but something got under my skin. Maybe it was just all about proving something: to others; to myself. Wondering just how far you can push yourself.

I began to run a little in the mornings before work. Just around the streets in the village in which I live. After building it up through regular short runs I took a deep breath and signed up for the Leeds 10k. Because If I can run 5K, I can run 10. Right? But more of that later.

Although I am not a good runner, having a tendency to both turn the colour of a ripe tomato and unhelpfully need a wee within seconds of setting off, I got better. Very slowly.

Running has given me experiences and taken me places (literally and figuratively) that I never thought I would go.

I went to Denmark to take place in a Corporate 25K relay challenge with colleagues from the Nordics. I've stood on the starting line with thousands of people in front of me and thousands more behind. I have run a muddy obstacle course, getting cold, wet mud in places that a girl should never find such a substance. I have taken part in a virtual marathon organised through social media.

I have run early in the morning on a beautiful spring day, pounding silent streets. I have run in the sunlight. I have run in the miserable cold and rain. I have run alone and with friends.

Here's the thing: I don't love running. Sometimes I don't even like it. But something compels you to do it all the same. The night before I race, I usually decide I don't want to go. That I have no idea why I signed up for this ridiculous thing in the first place. I think of all the lovely things that I could be doing instead, like having a weekend lie-in or a full English breakfast with all the trimmings. Or wine. But fast forward to the end of the run and you are already thinking about the next race, pondering a faster time, the next distance.

When I run, I feel like life is big. Like it has more colour. I also often feel like I might be dying.

When I am running I am mindful. I notice things I wouldn't normally see. Become someone else.

There is power, there is freedom, in your feet.

I am no longer fat.

The day that I knew for sure I was no longer fat was 12th July 2015. I ran the Leeds 10K. All the way. I signed up for it in February, and my aim was simply to run all the way around the course and not need to walk even a little bit. I trained for it. I went running before work. I did parkruns. I got myself the proper gear to run in, including an expensive pair of trainers just for my personal running style (I over pronate if you're interested). I worked hard in the gym to build up my stamina and the strength in my legs. I ate the right kind of breakfast. I got myself a gang of cheerleaders.

And I ran it. All the way. Every single step. I will confess to nearly shedding a tear as I crossed that finish line.

I was slow when compared to many running the course. I completed it in one hour, eleven minutes and eighteen seconds. I'm fairly sure that they were the best one hour, eleven minutes and eighteen seconds of my life until that point. It took about a further five minutes before I was criticising my own time and planning for how I could reduce it to under 60 minutes the next time around.

Here's the strange thing: whilst running the race I was counting down the minutes until it was over. I was desperate for it to be done. But I loved every minute of it too. I still can't quite reconcile those conflicting feelings. I think that running will always be a love / hate relationship for me. I will never like the process, but I am grateful for what it has given me.

When it comes to exercise there is a saying that I like: *run the race you are in*. It has two meanings to me. Firstly, it is about *this* race. It is about now. Not the next one or the last one but simply this run, right here, right now. Being totally present. The second meaning is about context; because good is different everywhere, and for everybody.

When you are running, or indeed doing any exercise, your real competitor is only yourself. You care about your performance and your time. That is why runners crave the elusive Personal Best. You might know that you can't compete with the elite runner, but you can be good for you, in your context and with your resources. There is no point in comparing my time to the time of the fittest, fastest runner in the race. It is good to look to others for inspiration. But at the same time, don't worry too much about what they are doing. They are running *their* race while you are running yours.

Back to the day in question. I arrived into the city centre early. Only a few early runners were already around. Empty streets, later to be filled with runners and their supporters cheering the way.

Leaving my family to get some breakfast, I walked alone to the finish line looming over the Headrow. I couldn't quite imagine what it would be like to cross it, but I did not doubt that I could.

Based on my estimated time I was the last group to begin. As I set off amongst the crowd the atmosphere was amazing. A sea of runners and colours, streaming all around me. The sound of thousands of feet striking the pavements. The cheers of the spectators, increasing when they spotted their friend or relative. Hearing my own name when I was spotted by my family. Music blaring.

Along the route a steel band that had come to play at the half way point. A Brownie troop singing songs. An elderly man handing out Jelly Babies to those running past him. Runners whooping as they ran through a tunnel, the echoes bouncing back and back. The turnaround point, when you knew you were on the way home. The truck spraying water from a fire hose cooling you at three quarters of the way through. The very welcome wet sponges at 9K. And finally coming around the corner and seeing the finish point. The time, nearly eight minutes quicker than I had hoped for, ticking away at the top. Strangers cheering you on. Finally crossing over the line.

That run was the culmination of the last three and a half years. I knew that I was not fat any more, not really. The mirror told me so. I knew that I was not unhealthy or unfit but I needed to prove it. Not to anyone else, but just to myself.

Now I had my proof. I had a medal to hold in my hand if I ever needed to see it. Even the aching muscles the following day were part of the triumph.

Oh, and then I went out and drank a bucket full of wine.

The following week, I signed up for my next race. Because it was possible to run it quicker next time, of course.

Stepping it Up

Early in 2015, the personal training company aligned to my gym offered some free 30 minute taster session. I was at a loose end so I went along, did some stuff and about three hours later was still recovering on my sofa. I couldn't lift my arms over my head for two days. I think it's fair to say that the PT in question had clearly mistaken me for someone fitter than I in fact was.

I signed up for ten sessions. And then ten more. I've found it an invaluable activity for lots of reasons.

At the beginning I was truly awful. There were times when I wanted to sit down in the middle of the gym and cry. I never actually did so but there a couple of occasions where I had a little snivel in the shower to myself afterwards when no one was looking.

After that first session, bits of my body hurt that I didn't know even existed. When I went back for my second session, the conversation with Mark, my trainer, went something like this:

Me: My arm hurts from our last session. I think I've pulled a muscle. I need to take it easy today and not do any weights.

PT: Is it swollen?

Me: No.

PT: Is it red?

Me: No.

PT: Is it warm to the touch?

Me: No.

PT: There is absolutely nothing wrong with you. Stop moaning. If you had really done some damage to your muscles you would know about it. Stop complaining, and get your fat lazy backside out of that chair and into the gym. You won't get fit if you are complaining all the time. You are perfectly capable of lifting weights, so suck it up.*

*He didn't actually say all or probably most of these things. I reckon he might have been thinking them though. What he actually said was something far nicer. Something about seeing how we went on during the session and adapting it as necessary. And then he made me get onto the treadmill and run.

And the simple truth is that this is exactly what I needed. There will always be someone in your life, maybe even yourself, that will accept and excuse and tell you it is okay to go home and oh poor little you. Sometimes these are the same reasons that you put weight on in the first place.

I don't have a problem with motivating myself to exercise. I do something pretty much every day, usually at some awful hour of the morning previously reserved for the snooze button. But we all need a little help from time to time, and this was the thing that really moved it for me. The thing that showed me what I was capable of.

The (first) big one.

Ten miles. In a moment of madness, I signed up to a 10 mile run. Because if I can run 10K, I can run 10 miles, right?

As with every time you run a new distance or a new course, you don't know quite what to expect. How will your body feel? How big will those hills be? Can you really make it all of the way around?

There's something a little bit special about a big event. The atmosphere, the build-up, the anticipation. Feeling simply part of something. Something bigger than yourself.

I did not train well for it. A busy work schedule, badly timed holiday and a nasty cold, coupled with actually, a real dislike of running very far, meant I had not done anywhere near enough training as I should have done in preparation. But still, you turn up all the same.

The day dawned warm and sunny. An early start, off to the park and ride. Arriving at the event village, people everywhere. The biggest event I've attended so far.

The run was through York on the same day as the Yorkshire Marathon. Those hardy 26.2 mile folks went first with two thousand or so 10 milers setting off just afterwards. The course going straight through the historical city centre and then out into the Yorkshire country side, through country lanes and small villages. Marathon runners on the left, 10 milers on the right.

When I got to about mile six or so, by then very much towards the back of the 10 mile crowd, the two races merged into one course. The shout came up from behind that the first marathon runner was coming through. Shouts and cheers of encouragement all the way from every other runner. All in it together.

It was all going reasonably well until the worst thing that has happened to me on a run, happened. At the beginning of the race, we'd been told that there were water stations ever three miles. After an hour and a half or more of running, I was tired and I was running out of energy despite all the Jelly Babies I'd consumed along the way. And then, a water station. The third one. And in the distance, a few hundred yards past the water station, a yellow distance marker. Mile nine. There was only one more mile to go. That wasn't so bad. I could manage one more mile surely. So I drank from the water station and then I ran and I thought I was nearly home. Only as I got nearer to the flag, it didn't look all that much like a number nine. In fact, the closer I got, the more it looked very much like a number eight. Dawning realisation. Not one more mile left, but two.

I might* have said a very, very rude word.

All I really wanted to do was run all the way and come in under two hours. I achieved both, partially through the kindness of strangers. The last part of this run was a bloody great big hill. At the bottom, a school band was playing - drums banging, trumpets, well, trumping. Just, a few more hundred yards. Just me and one girl, next to each other. A total stranger, yet in it together. She would inch ahead, and then I would. Both of us pushing up that hill together, pushing each other, both heaving for breath. The 'you are nearly there' shouts actually true this time. Every step, now painful. Each breath harder to take.

And there it was. The finish line. The time clock showing me one hour and 59 minutes.

Target achieved.

*Did. Very loudly. I would like to apologise about that to anyone who heard it.

So that's my story. How I put it on, what I have spent the last four years doing, and how I found a new life and a new me along the way. No different to a dozen or so other stories that you have read or watched perhaps.

You learn a lot about yourself when you lose weight. Even more when you try and get fit. Some good learnings, some more difficult. As I said right at the beginning, the reason why I put pen to paper to write this little book was just to see if any of those things that I have learned along the way could be helpful to someone else.

So the next few chapters are about practical stuff. Advice. Tips. Things to try. Both weight loss and exercise based.

In no particular order, here are my main learnings from the last few years, whether it is weight loss of fitness you are trying to achieve.

1. The reasons that you got overweight or unfit in the first place are multifactorial. So therefore the solution needs to be too. There isn't just one thing that you will need to do, one change you will need to make. This problem will have to be tackled on many levels.

2. Run the race you are in. There is no point comparing yourself to others. Whether that is someone in an actual race who can run faster or for longer, or just someone else in a slimming class who lost a pound more than you did. Your only competition is yourself. Just aim to be better than you used to be, better than you were yesterday.

3. Resist lots of advice. I mean, apart from mine of course. There is so much information out there on different diets and eating plans. Different fitness regimes. Exercises to fire up your metabolic rate. 5 ways to shift your stubborn belly fat. Books, magazines, blogs, articles. Juice cleanses, detox plans, 5:2, Weightwatchers, Slimming World, Atkins, protein shakes. Are you beach body ready? It goes on and on. There is no miracle cure. There is no one size fits all solution. If there was, there

would be no diet industry. We'd all just go on a diet, lose the weight and never struggle ever again. The world would all be skinny.

4. Weight loss is both terribly hard, and incredibly simple. The belief that you can lose it, is hard. Sticking to it when you really want a curry followed by a family size bag of Maltesers, is hard. Exercise, especially at the start, is very hard. Fighting against years of failures, against all the people who don't believe you are going to do it this time, or would secretly like to see you fail, is hard.

5. Losing weight actually isn't hard to do – in theory at least. East less crap. Drink more water. Get plenty of sleep. Move more – as much as you can. Stay away from processed junk that does nothing good for your body. Eat less sugar and refined stuff. Eat lots and lots of protein. Read my later chapter and follow some of the tips. Set yourself a clearly measurable goal. And go for it.

6. Diets fail and exercise programmes fail because people give up. And giving up is a mental process, just like weight loss is to a large extent. The most important thing you can do, is believe.

And so to the more detailed advice. First up: weight loss.

How I did it.

When people find out that you lost a lot of weight, they are often interested in how you did it. Only I find that when I simply tell them that I ate less crap and got off the sofa more, it isn't all that welcome. People want to know how you went on some fabulous plan that they can also follow or read some miracle book that they can order from Amazon. They don't want to know that you get up a 5.30am every morning to work your ass off in the gym and rarely eat many of my favourite foods.

But there are no quick fixes or simple solutions. So just in case you want to try it and see if it works for you, here is what I did, in no particular order. Please note: this is not a diet. This is a lifestyle, a way of being. A way of eating and being that I can live with for the rest of my life. There is simply no other way to think about it if you want a long term solution.

First things first. I am not telling you that you should do it my way. I am not an expert in the field or a qualified nutritionist. I am just someone who has been there and tried things and learned what worked for them along the way, and what didn't work too.

Here goes......

Watch diet and low fat branded products. Many brands have a low calorie or low fat version of a (probably) tastier product. They tend to fall into two categories (or sometimes both) in my experience. The first is that they are low in taste as well as low in other stuff. The other is that the fat and the calories are replaced with a chemical storm of nastiness that won't help you in the long term. Sometimes, the low fat versions have more calories in than the original product. So stop eating these and replace it with cleaner food.

Don't be scared of fats. For years, fats were thought of as bad and something to be avoided. But there are good fats and bad fats. Good fats are Olive Oil, natural Greek Yoghurt, avocado, oily fish and nuts like almonds and walnuts. Bad fats are the obvious ones. Those found in fast foods or ready meals. Include the former in your diet, definitely. The rest, not so much.

Next suggestion. Make it a regular habit to read the labels on what you eat. So much food that is portrayed as healthy is anything but. Take breakfast cereal. Many of them are heaving with sugar and other things that are really sugar by another name. We all know that the chocolate or frosted versions probably aren't good for the waistline, but some that look healthy like muesli or granola are not much better. A bowl full of that, plus the milk and a coffee or two, and you will easily be racking up over 500 calories for your breakfast. Smoothies, fruit juices, even your favourite coffee can be loaded with invisible calories. Understand what you are eating before you actually eat it. If you still want it, fine, go ahead. But eat it from a position of being informed.

Limit your fizzy drinks. Yes, even the diet versions. The full fat versions are truly awful. Full of sugar and calories that have no nutritional value at all, cause insulin spikes and are also often full of caffeine too which will have a negative impact on your sleep. Even the zero calorie versions can be full of chemicals, and their sweetness might just encourage you to eat other sweet food. Or they have lots of caffeine which equally isn't helpful in your diet. Drink water instead. It is not as nice, but it is hugely important for weight loss. As well as the fact it has no calories, fat or other unhelpful stuff, it is good for your skin and helps flush your system through. Drink plenty. 2 litres a day minimum. And yes, you will go to the toilet a whole heck of a lot.

Eat little and often. Keep your metabolism working. 10% of the calories you burn every day are just from your body digesting food. The technical term is the 'thermal effect of feeding'. Don't skip meals, especially breakfast. That cliché is most definitely true.

When it comes to weight loss, calorie counting is some of it, but not all of it. If you are a woman and you want to lose weight at a sensible rate then you should be aiming for about 1500 calories a day. But this still won't work if they are rubbish calories that lack nutritional value or other stuff that is going to help shift the pounds. There is a big difference between 1500 calories of chocolate and 1500 calories of vegetables, so don't kid yourself.

Eat protein. Lots and lots of protein. For all the reading I have done about weight loss, and all the diets I have tried – both sensible and ridiculous – the importance and the power of protein had really passed me by. In early 2015 I found that my weight was stuck, even though I was eating fewer calories than I was burning off. A review of my diet with my trainer found it to be too high in fruit (including all the sugar within it) and lacking in protein. Eating the same calories but swapping other foods for ones high in protein made a massive difference. It also helps build lean muscle so this change is even more important if you are exercising too. More muscle means that your body burns more calories at rest - even when you are sitting on the sofa. And if you are wondering ladies, you will not end up looking like Arnie. Our bodies just aren't built what way. So go lift something heavy.

Get plenty of sleep. Tiredness can lead to weight gain and disordered eating. Go to bed earlier than you usually do, turn off your devices and don't fall asleep in front of the TV. Try and keep a good routine of going to bed and getting up at a similar time.

Eat what you fancy in moderation. I typically follow an 80-20 rule. 80% of the time I am good and disciplined, but every so often, usually on holiday or special occasions, I eat what the hell I want. If you think that you have on average 21 main meals a week, it will not hurt you terribly if three of these meals are a little off plan. This advice will work for some people, not others. For me, I needed it. I eat really well five days a week, and at weekends I am much more relaxed. If I want wine on a Friday night, I have it. I will go out to dinner and have a dessert. Occasionally, a cake might appear in my Saturday afternoon. But I never skip my weekend exercise, and I always get straight back on it on Monday morning. For some, this is a slippery slope to bad habits, but if can get your head in the right place, it is a much easier way to live than trying to stick constantly to some sort of diet plan. I am, without fail, two pounds heavier on a Monday morning than a Friday morning. I can live with that. Balance in all things.

Most people eat useless calories. In my bigger days I was an orange juice fiend and I was probably taking in over 300 calories a day from juice alone. So I switched juice to something that was a treat rather than an everyday occurrence. I missed it for a few weeks, but now I barely drink it at all. So look at where you are taking in unnecessary calories, empty calories. And take them out of your diet, one at a time.

Record what you eat. All of it. Whether you use an App or a diary, write down everything you eat and every calorie that you consume *as you eat them*. If you try and remember what you ate at the end of the day, you will not remember all of it. This process will focus your mind and help you deal with the reality of what you eat. This will not work if you are not truthful. And if you are not truthful, the only person you are lying to is yourself.

Exercise is important. It will speed up your efforts and make you feel better about yourself, and it will help you tone. But you can't exercise away a bad diet. What you weigh is about 80% what you eat and 20% what exercise you do. But do the exercise anyway. More about that later.

Find someone or something to inspire you. I have a fitness inspiration board on Pinterest. I am also a big fan of the TV programme *Obese, A Year to Save My Life.* I watch it over and over, rooting for the people who are working so hard to make changes in their life, most of them fighting a battle harder than the one I have faced. It doesn't matter what it is, just find something to help you along the path when you are having a bad day.

You will probably have heard of 'clean' eating. What does this really mean? Simple really. It is about eating food as close to its natural state as possible. Fresh, raw, unprocessed. The less your food is processed and the less it is added to or changed, the healthier it will be for you. So ditch the ready meals and the Trans fats (which will probably show as 'hydrogenated fat' on a nutrition label), stay away from processed junk, whatever the calorie count. The more processed something is, whether it is white bread or microwave ready meal, the more additives, preservatives and chemicals there will be in it. The cleaner your food is, the closer to its natural state, the better it will be for your body, your mind, and ultimately, your weight. I'm not suggesting you need to start a juice diet (I'm really, really not) but more veg, more brown bread too (or better still Rye), more green stuff…. This is the way not just to weight loss, but health.

Don't drink stuff with lots of caffeine in after 2pm. It lasts for ages in your system, and even at 2pm it can impact negatively on your ability to sleep that night.

Beware of 'healthy' food. Some of it is anything but. Even the genuinely good stuff needs moderation. Take fruit. Good for you, right? One of your five a day, contains lots of vitamins and also contributes to the fluid intake you need. But it's also often full of sugar and it doesn't fill you up for long. As I said earlier, when it comes to all food, especially those touted as healthy options, always read the label to make sure that they are as healthy as they say they are.

Weigh yourself as often as you need to – do whatever works for you. Some people will say you shouldn't weigh yourself more than once a week. I weigh myself every day. It is how I keep myself on track. It is no surprise that my slow weight creep took place during years where I didn't own a pair of scales. It helps me to keep an eye on it and see what makes it fluctuate, for good or for bad. So on this one make up your own rules.

You will have heard people say aim for 2lb of weight loss a week. There's a reason for that. Firstly, it is sustainable. Secondly, if you lose more than that then you are not really losing weight but muscle and other generally helpful stuff to your body. To lose 2lb a week you need to reduce your overall calorie consumption by 500 calories per day. Your food diary will tell you what you are currently eating, the rest is just mathematics.

Alcohol. Now this is probably unwelcome news, but booze is pretty disastrous for weight loss. It is full of sugar and empty calories. It increases your appetite and makes you more likely to make poor food choices, especially when you've had a few. If you want to get lean you will have to reduce what you drink. Possibly a lot. Time to stick to the weekly guidelines as an absolute maximum. Sorry about that.

What all of this advice boils down to is mostly this: eat less crap and move around more.

Easy to say, a whole lot less easy to do perhaps.

So rather than the simplistic 'eat less, move more' mantra I would suggest this instead; eat well and move plenty.

You don't need me to tell you what is good food and bad food. For the most part that is obvious. It isn't a diet sheet that people need, it is something else.

But if you are reading this book and you want to lose weight, I reckon you already know a lot of what is written here. You have lived it. There's no rocket science or thought leadership here. Just sensible advice that you can get from anywhere.

So here's a thought: if you already know it, why haven't you done it?

Stuff to know about losing weight that no one ever tells you.

Number One: *Everybody has an opinion about it.*

When I was getting fatter and fatter, no one said anything. It's a taboo subject after all. But the same doesn't seem to apply when your weight is going the other way. Everyone has an opinion on how you should do it. Plenty of people think that it is just fine to tell you that it is time to stop. A couple of people felt it necessary to tell me recently that I was getting too thin in the face and that I wasn't looking so hot. I don't listen to these people. None of them felt the need to say anything when I was eating my way to diabetes and heart disease, so I pay no heed now.

The most important opinion is my own. Listen to your inner voice before you listen to other people's opinions – most of which are only that. Their opinion. They have not walked a mile in your shoes.

Number Two: *Some people will have an issue with it.*

When you are fat, you have a persona. Sometimes, you fulfil a certain role for other people or within a group. Is it a co-incidence that when I lost a lot of weight some people were not around in my life anymore or upped the sarcastic jokes? The truth is I don't really know. But I do know that some people changed towards me. This is sad, for them. It is not your problem so give not one single flying fuck.

Number Three: *If you are a woman*, your boobs will disappear.*

That is all I have to say about that.

Number Four: *Everyone will want to know how you did it.*

But they will not want to know that you just got off your arse more and ate less junk food. Most people want something more interesting than that.

Number Five. *Losing weight is one thing. Keeping it off is another.*

For lots of overweight people food represents something. Food is a friend. Food makes you feel better. Food is a coping mechanism. At the very least it is something hugely enjoyable even if its consequences are not. Its absence, keenly felt. So something has to fill the gap. It isn't unusual for gastric bypass patients who can no longer eat in the quantities that they did before surgery to fall victim to other addictions. Many dieters go on to regain the weight that they have lost. And there is no easy fix for this problem either.

This may also apply to a man. I have no personal experience through which I can confirm or deny this.

In my experience, people who are overweight often tell themselves lies about being overweight. There's a reason for it. It is nice. It is far more pleasant to tell yourself a sequence of soothing, comforting fibs, than face the cold, hard, obese truth.

There is a thing that goes on in our brain called cognitive dissonance. Our brains naturally do not like to hold two contradictory beliefs or ideas at the same time. We strive for consistency, and where there is none, we try and create it. We try to bring our beliefs and our everyday reality closer together. So it goes a bit like this: I want to lose weight, and I know that I will need to eat less chocolate for that to happen, but I also want to eat the chocolate, so chocolate can't be all that bad especially if I only have a little bit and anyway I am going to the gym tomorrow so I will just work really hard when I am there and that will balance it all out and there aren't even that many calories in it anyway because it is made of milk and that comes from cows and they eat grass so it is practically one of my five a day anyway so for goodness sake PASS ME THE CHOCOLATE NOW. I'm exaggerating a little with the example obviously, but the brain thing is true.

We engage in this stuff all the time when we are trying to lose some weight. Recently I went to a BBQ with a friend who is trying to diet. There was a mountain of food. All of it nice, none of it healthy. There were crisps and popcorn and cake and sausage rolls and dips and wine and pizza and wine and garlic bread and wine. And some wine too. This was before they even lit the BBQ. I knew in advance I was going to struggle to eat well so I took some chicken and put it on the BBQ myself. It didn't keep me away from the crisps, but it was a better choice than the hot-dogs. My friend indulged. She ate burgers and hot-dogs and crisps and more crisps and another hot-dog and some of my chicken and some more of the crisps, and washed it down with a load of beer. Later on, she was hungry again. Hunting for a snack, she said to me *"It isn't surprising I'm hungry, I didn't really eat anything today"*. And the most interesting thing about this statement is that she absolutely believed it. She didn't want to remember all the high fat food that she had consumed and so she minimised it to herself. This is reason for the recommendation to keep a food diary. And not just at the end of the day but meal by meal– because later you will conveniently forget what you put in your mouth.

Many of us are secret eaters. Sometimes, we are just hiding what we eat from others. Chocolate wrappers hidden at the bottom of the bin, biscuits replaced before anyone notices they are missing, blaming someone else (you wouldn't believe the food that my step-son eats when he comes to visit….). But sometimes the person we are hiding the secret from is simply ourselves.

If you are reading this book and you are overweight then there is a chance that you too are engaging in a spot of truth distortion. We all do it.

Here are the lies I used to tell myself:

Lie: I might be in a large dress size, but I carry it well.

Truth: *I didn't carry it well at all. There is rarely such a thing.*

Lie: I only wear a size 22 because I like my clothes to be loose fitting.

Truth: *I wore a size 22 because it fitted me and the next size down didn't.*

Lie: I don't eat all that much, it isn't fair.

Truth: *If you call devouring family size bags of chocolate every evening not eating much, then I didn't eat much. Weight is a simple formula. Eat more calories than you burn off on a regular basis and you will put weight on.*

Lie   Lots of the food I eat isn't even that bad for you.

Truth   *In moderation, yes. Orange juice, your particular favourite, isn't bad for you. It has vitamins and stuff. But not a litre a day.*

Lie   I don't have time to exercise.

Truth	*Rubbish. Anyone who wants to find time to exercise, can find time to exercise. Watch less garbage on the TV. Get up earlier. You had time to go to the pub, so you had time to exercise. Prioritise.*
Lie	I eat healthy food. I don't know why I am fat.
Truth	*I was known to eat the occasional banana or tomato. But that does not balance out a whole tub of Ben and Jerry's ice cream. Sadly.*
Lie	It's not fair.
Truth	*It is what it is.*

And finally, the biggest lie of all.

Lie:	I can't lose weight. I've tried. It doesn't work.
Truth:	*Like hell you tried. Eating lettuce for two days and then sulking when you hadn't dropped four dress sizes is not trying to lose weight. Anybody can lose weight. Weight is a simple mathematical formula of food in versus energy burned off. But it is bloody hard work and needs much commitment.*

I'm not suggesting that everyone who is overweight is deliberately lying to themselves and others. Because beneath all of these lies is a belief. I genuinely believed all of these things, and more. If you can change your belief you can change everything, anything. That voice in your head that says you can't do this is a liar.

There is another thing about how the brain works which is relevant to losing weight. It's called confirmation bias. Put simply this is the tendency for us to look to confirm what we already believe. So if we believe that we are not really all that fat and we don't eat all that badly, we will look everywhere for information to support that viewpoint. Every banana will be carefully recalled, every family size bag of chocolate buttons most definitely forgotten. A single but not very sweaty trip the gym taken as proof that it's not all my fault, it must be my genes, my slow metabolic rate, the unfairness of it all.

Our memories are selective. The more entrenched the belief, the tighter we hold onto it. Even being presented with evidence makes no difference at all. All the sweet wrappers in the world won't change our minds.

When people say 'I can't lose weight', what they usually mean is that they believe this to be true; they have tried it, failed, and so are taking this as even more proof, then believed it all the more.

Part one of my theory of dieting is this. Like most change, it all begins with self-awareness and the dismantling of denial. Like the alcoholic who doesn't think they have a drink problem, you won't address your eating problems until you truly face them – or have your own moment. I believe that many overweight people only understand their weight on a surface level. Just like I did; you know you have a problem, but you minimise it, deny it, make it more palatable to live with.

Getting up close and personal with the truth is where the change begins. And the truth, beings in the scales.

So think about those lies that you tell yourself. If you knew that they weren't true, what would you do?

Boiling Frogs

As well as women's magazines, I also love a weight loss TV programme. I watch them all. Fat Families, Secret Eaters, My 600lbs life, Fat the Fight of My Life. You name it, it's on series link.

As is the way with a lot of reality TV, the most extreme examples are often featured. The biggest, fattest possible people eating the biggest possible portions. It is easy to watch one of these programmes, to see someone who is super morbidly obese and wonder how they got there, how they allowed themselves to get quite that fat.

I know the answer to that question.

One mouthful of food at a time.

Have you heard about the story of the boiling frog? Apparently, if you put a frog in a pan of boiling water it will jump out. Somewhat unsurprisingly perhaps. However, if you were so cruel as to put a frog in a pan of cold water and then slowly heat it up, the frog is unable to perceive the changes in temperature and will simply sit there until they are cooked all the way through. And hence, very dead. Trust, me this is a real theory. Honest. Look it up on Wikipedia. It is used to illustrate how people just often aren't aware of gradual creeping changes because of how slowly they occur.

That is weight gain right there. Because it's just one biscuit, right? And one takeaway won't hurt. There are only 200 calories in the whole packet. Those leftovers in the fridge need eating up.

The problem with weight gain is how slowly it takes place. You only really notice when you go up a size in clothes, or you are suddenly no longer able to do something.

If you put on ten stone overnight and tomorrow morning found yourself unable to tie your own shoe laces, get out of a chair without help, or climb the stairs without pausing for breath, you would be horrified. If in the space of a week you went from a size 8 in Top Shop to the plus size store, you would very quickly do something about it. You'd be on a diet and down the gym.

But it doesn't happen like that. The water slowly heats up and you don't even notice until it is too late and poor old Kermit is cooked all the way through.

For me, I gave up wearing anything but trousers. Skirts, dresses, shorts and the like were out. Then I stopped wearing high heels to work because my knees wouldn't take it. Then I gave up wearing heels at all. I gave up wearing swimming costumes on the beach, opting instead opting for the big girl's friend; the cover-all maxi dress. Some things I didn't even know I had given up. Take crossing your legs. I didn't realise that I hadn't been able to cross my legs at the knee for years until I could again!

And so on, and so on.

One mouthful at a time.

Enablers and Detractors

If you want to lose weight then there is an important but uncomfortable issue that you may need to confront.

Who around you is helping you to eat? And who around you is not helping you to make the changes that you want to make, that you *need* to make? The people around you can have either a positive or negative impact on your weight loss journey. I've experienced some of the negative, and a fair few folks with an opinion too.

First things first: you are 100% responsible for every single thing that you put in your mouth – every single food choice you make. Believing otherwise is the key to either never losing weight or putting it all back on again. There are some things that make sticking to a diet harder. For me it's travelling with work, conferences or training courses where there are biscuits at every break, or just simply, the weekends. But you are still responsible for all of the choices that you make.

Now, there is always a choice. *Your* choice. Even if that choice is between two really crappy things, or two things that you really want but contradict each other. Like the desire to be both thin but eat all the food you want to eat. But it is still your choice, every time.

Only sometimes there are people around you who are either actively encouraging you to make bad choices or enabling you to make them. When I lost weight, I found that other people shared their own stories with me; stories of both success and failure. I've heard plenty of examples of enablers and detractors, as well as experiencing my own share too.

Some people are out and out feeders. You may well have seen the slightly odd TV programmes. Often feeders are men who like a larger lady, they are actively engaged in a feeding relationship. Weird? Maybe. But it is only an extreme version of something that is often much more subtle.

It might be someone telling you that you look beautiful when you are overweight, because they don't want to hurt your feelings by telling you the truth. It might equally be someone who you thought would be there for you, who is instead silent just when you begin to make changes. It might be someone who is also overweight, who wants you to stay just as you are because then they don't have to face their own issues. It might be an insecure partner filling your plate with giant portions, telling you that he likes you 'just the way you are'. It may be someone who uses food to show their love.

Whichever category they fall into there is one similarity. This is their issue. Not yours. As the saying goes, you can't change someone else, you can only change the way you react to them.

If you have an enabler or a detractor in your life, you will have to face up to it and deal with it in whatever way is most appropriate for you.

I have a rule about those that have an opinion on my weight loss. If the person sharing their views also had a well-intentioned conversation with me about my weight gain, when I was obese and heading in the direction of all sorts of serious health conditions, I will listen to what they have to say. If they didn't then I will take no notice.

And for the record, this adds up to precisely no people.

For a final word on this subject I'm going to hand over to my friend, Julie Drybrough, who wrote this:

Who is around when we step into what radiates and inspires us? Who can bear to look at us when we are beautiful? Who can stand with us, without snide comment or sniping? Just like who can stand with us when we are ugly and weak and scared and can hold our beauty for us for a while. Some can do both. Some cannot. Forgive the silence. In that, they are having their own struggle. It may show up as bitchiness or rejection. This is about your, your choices, your beautiful self. Not anyone else.

Rubbish the media tells you

As I've already confessed, I am partial to a women's magazine or three.

Women's magazines feature a lot of weight loss articles. Usually they are inspirational stories of people who have lost a whole heap of weight, and details of how they did it. You can be sure that it will include a 'what she ate before' and 'what she eats now' sidebar. The before section will usually indicate that this particular former fatty lived on the likes of chocolate digestives, takeaways and fried food, all washed down with full fat Coke. Now of course they have seen the light and live on salad, protein, and snack on nuts and the like. *(Note to Reader: I don't know about you but the definition of 'snack' when it comes to healthy eating isn't my definition of a snack. To me, a snack is a Kit Kat. Or a sausage roll. Or bag of crisps. Nuts and seeds..... not so much.)*

Am I the only one who looks at the 'before' diet and wants to eat all of it?

Wherever you look in a magazine of this type, there is someone trying to sell you a diet or evangelise a particular approach. Most of them are of the quick fix variety. Lose seven pounds before your holidays on our detox diet! Beat the bloat. Burn that belly fat. How to get a thigh gap, fast! Get beach body ready! And so on.

I'm going to suggest there has been more utter garbage written about weight loss than any other subject in the history of man. Except possibly Human Resources (which is what I do when I'm not in the gym).

It isn't limited to magazines either. Social media is full of it too. In that space, everything seems to start with a number. 5 ways to do this. 7 absolute ways to do something else.

Photoshopped models. Impossible ideals. Images, everywhere.

We are constantly bombarded with so-called "ideal" images that simply do not represent the average person. But we are influenced by them all the same.

They sell us a fantasy. A fallacy.

There are some things that you just can't change. Your genetics for one. Your body type for another. Some of the fat you have and where you store it is genetically determined and there is almost nothing you can do about it.

Going back to the magazines for a moment. Some of the plans they peddle come with a few exercises you can do in the comfort of your own bedroom. Often whilst holding a can of beans just in case you don't have any free weights. Well I'm here to tell you that a few bicep curls or a handful of tricep dips off the side of the bed are going to do pretty much nothing at all. As I write this chapter, I've been weight lifting several times a week for more than a year. I Zumba. I swim. I run. I ride my bike. I do weight training. And I still have bingo wings, a very wobbly bottom, and more cellulite than I care to look at. I'm sorry to be the bearer of bad news, but getting toned is a long, long process. I don't know how long, because I haven't done it yet. It may never happen for me, given how I previously stretched my skin further than what should be considered reasonable.

There are no quick fixes. No matter what the latest guru or carefully edited celebrity tells you.

More rubbish about weight loss

First things first. Most 'diets' don't work. Many diets that become popularised in the press or are followed by celebrities don't even have any conclusive evidence that they work.

The diet industry continues to expand and profit whilst dangling the promise of miracle weight loss solutions but at the same time the obesity crisis is escalating.

Whether it is 5:2, Cayenne Pepper, juice cleanses, Atkins, Paleo, or a diet based on your blood type, the simple truth is that if you create a calorie deficit then weight loss should result. Whether it is desirable weight loss is however an entirely different thing.

Take the Atkins diet. This is all about reducing or eliminating carbs from your diet. The problem with this approach is that carbs are your bodies preferred source of energy. We need them. So if you follow Atkins to the letter then you are missing an important element of your nutritional requirements. Even worse, Atkins isn't that healthy (think about all that meat and eggs) and what you are going to lose from your body is not fat but lean muscle mass – the opposite of what you really want.

Many diets can help you achieve short term weight loss. This is fine if this is your goal. But many of them are also deficient in the nutrients that the body really needs which is definitely not good long term. Many of them are also very boring, which leads to dieters falling off the wagon.

The big problem with many diets is that they fail completely to address the reason that someone put weight on in the first place. They deal only with the symptoms of weight loss and not the cause.

Very low calorie diets are not the answer (some good news at long last!). They might lead to short term rapid weight loss but they have a terrible impact on the body. Anything less than 1000Kcal per day will reduce weight but, like the Atkins diet, it will come from water and lean tissue. To compensate for what it perceives as a threat the body will slow down. Weight loss will soon plateau. Even worse, if you begin eating normally again the body will perceive it as a binge and store the excess as fat even if it was originally weight lost from lean tissue.

Some approaches work well for some people. Take weight loss groups. For some, the peer support and the weekly weigh-in really help them along the way. Others hate the idea of groups. But there are a few good things about this sort of approach to weight loss – primarily that they can help to re-educate people about healthy portion sizes and good food choices. So although they didn't work for me personally, they are still definitely worth a try.

In terms of evaluating a potential diet (if you must call it such a thing):

If a diet requires you to reduce daily calories to something daft like 500 a day, it is a fad diet.

If a diet requires you to cut out entire food groups (unless it is related to your medical history), it is a probably a fad diet.

If a diet requires you to eat or drink some very strange concoctions and nothing else at all, it is probably a fad diet.

If a diet includes or recommends exercise, includes all food groups in balance, focusing on healthy eating above anything, and has a sensible calorie intake that provides you with enough energy, then it is probably a reasonable approach to take. And if it can point to some evidence, then all the better.

Stuff to watch out for......

Diet programmes that are busy selling you their shakes, their ready meals, their snack bars. Often meal replacements are expensive, taste dodgy and fail to support long term healthy eating changes.

Diets that are expensive to do and require all manner of complicated and expensive ingredients. You just don't need them to lose weight safely and effectively.

Diets that promise very high weight loss in a short period of time – no diet can deliver this in an effective way that will lead to long term sustainability.

Diets that exclude certain food groups as these may well mean you are not getting your full complement of vitamins, minerals and nutrients.

Diets that ask you to eat lots of one particular food, like grapefruit or cabbage soup. You will miss out on vital elements of a healthy diet, it is hellishly boring and, contrary to the myths, there are no foods that burn fat!

Diets that are endorsed by a celebrity. Always remember that they have been paid to do it!

Diets that lack any evidence. Like, at all. And the one thing that absolutely does not amount to evidence, is a snap-shot case study of one or two individuals saying that they have lost weight doing it.

Instead what really works is in fact obvious, only perhaps not as interesting or quick or easy to advertise. And definitely not the celebrity endorsed, accompanying Boxing Day DVD type approach. Simply put, it's clean eating, long term changes, good nutrition and regular exercise.

Bugger.

I have just one more thing to say about diets. *There will be another one along in a minute.* Another diet programme, another celebrity endorsement, another promise of a miracle. And it won't be any different to the last one. And nor will the outcome.

Exercise

And talking of exercise......

First of all, the good news. Or the bad news, depending on your point of view.

Exercise doesn't make you thin.

Exercise supports weight loss, helps to maintain weight loss, and helps you tone. But by itself, it will not help you get skinny, if that's your goal.

Weight loss is about 80% what you eat and about 20% what you do.

It does help do lots of other stuff though. Reduces the risk of a whole load of not so nice diseases and improves your cardiovascular health. Reduces cholesterol and blood pressure. It's good for your psychological health too. The list of reasons why you should exercise could go on for pages. So it does need to be part of the programme.

But you can't out exercise a shitty diet. If you eat a doughnut, you can't run off the doughnut. Sad but true. Otherwise believe me, I would do a lot more running.

My exercise journey began in my living room. A 10 minute fat burner DVD. 10 minutes for your bum, 10 minutes for your arms and so on. I started with the thigh set given that it was one of my problem areas (and sadly, still is). A shouty and much toned American woman instructing me robustly to squat and lunge. It was pretty awful. It was even more awful an hour later when I drove to work and realised I couldn't get out of the car.

But I was moving.

So my advice is simply this: move your body. In whatever way floats your boat. 3-5 times a week, for at least 30 minutes. Swim, run, walk, Zumba, weight train, box, cycle, row...

Simply move, and often.

If you start to enjoy it, get serious about it, make it part of your life, then there are all sorts of options about how you move it forward. The most important thing to do though, is find something that you enjoy. At least a little bit.

So here is my advice for exercise.......

Sign up for an event even if you aren't sure if you can do it. Do a Race for Life, book a class you have never taken, go to a boot camp in the park. You might do really well or you might be dead last. But it is better to regret trying something than regret doing nothing at all. And you never know, you might just rock it. And as they say in running circles, *dead last is better than did not finish, which is better than did not start.*

Keep your eye on sites like Groupon. Sometimes their offers include fitness classes or outdoor boot camps, so it is a handy way of trying something out without a big expense until you are sure you like it.

Gym gear. It might feel like an additional expense, but you do need some basics. If you are a woman, then a well-fitting and supportive sports bra is a must. So is a good pair of trainers, whatever your gender.

Exercise with someone else. I tried both parkrun and Sweatshop when I was getting into running – more about both of them later.

It isn't all about going to the gym or doing loads of cardio either. All activity is good. And they might be clichés but taking the stairs rather than the lift, walking instead of taking the car.... Building activity into your daily life rather than sitting on the sofa is what counts.

Find your exercise thing. Lots of people will tell you running is awesome. Others will wax lyrical about the joys of cycling, weight lifting or Pilates. Which is usually what they like and what has worked for them. A good friend of mine recently took up boxing and found an unexpected passion. Another friend is a Zumba Queen. So try different stuff until you find the thing that you like. Because the more you enjoy it, the more likely you are to stick to it.

Whatever it is you chose to do, make sure it is doable for you and your lifestyle. The reason that lots of people give up on exercise is that what they have set out to do feels too big, too much of a change or burden.

Start small, start simple and then build.

Things that happen when you begin to exercise that you might not be expecting

You will get very keen on sports clothing and will suddenly be prepared to spend money previously dedicated to shoes and handbags on swanky looking gym wear.

You will feel like you are spending half your life washing this swanky looking gym wear.

You will learn a whole new terminology and embrace your inner geek. Who knew what over-pronating was until you went for an analysis of your running style?

Some of your other not-so-healthy habits disappear along the way with very little awareness, as your exercise and improved lifestyle spills out into other parts of your life. I gave up smoking once I began running and I didn't even notice.

You will get called boring by friends and family who aren't interested in exercise, when you don't order a dessert, only have the one glass of wine, and so on. You won't even care that much.

You will sleep like a baby.

You will begin to care about the elusive Personal Best. Quite a bit, actually.

You will realise it is entirely possible to get stuck in a sports bra. (Probably just one for the girls this point).

You will be willing to get up in the morning to do strange things like go to a parkrun, even if it means leaving a nice warm bed.

There are few better feelings than realising your body can do something that it couldn't do just a few weeks ago.

It gets seriously addictive.

The Truth

Now that the lies, cognitive distortions and stuff and nonsense are out of the way, here are the truths about a weight loss and fitness journey as I have personally found them.

It will be hard work. But then again, so is being fat.

It will take a long time. Longer than you think. There are no sustainable quick fixes.

You are capable of more than you ever thought you could be.

Sometimes, you will have a bad day or a bad week. You will fall back into bad habits. You might even binge a little. But you can continue along the path all the same.

Exercise hurts. In the beginning, it hurts a lot. But you can get to like those aches and pains in a strange sort of way, as they are a symbol that you are changing who you used to be.

There will be times when you think you cannot go on. Trust me, you can.

If you eat what you have always eaten, you will weigh what you have always weighed or, frankly, a lot more.

You will never regret it.

Some bits of your skin will never go back to how you would like them to be. That sucks, to be honest.

Belief is everything.

It took years to put it on so you can't expect it to come off in a few weeks. One pound at a time: keep your eyes on the prize.

It is never too late to make this change.

Buying new clothes in the next size down is one of the best feelings in the world.

The only person who can do this is you.

You will have to give up some of the foods that you love. You will miss them a little, but it is far outweighed by what you get in return.

Excuses don't burn calories. Dieting alone isn't enough. You need to exercise too.

No matter how busy you think you are, you have time for exercise. You just have to want to make the time.

You will start to enjoy exercise.

You will have bad days. But this isn't a reason to give up. Just start again tomorrow.

You are totally in charge of your own perspective.

You are not trapped by your weight, neither are you defined by it. You are only trapped by your own attitude towards it.

And the most important truth of all. *It will be worth it.*

There is one other quote that I use all the time. It applies to work, weight loss, exercise, life in general. *If you want to badly enough, you will find a way. If not, you will find an excuse.* This is one of the most truthful things anyone has ever said (or turned into a motivational poster). If you meet someone who allegedly wants to exercise but hasn't got round to it or keeps finding barriers, they will typically give you a list of reasons why not. The classes are at the same time I have to put the kids to bed, I don't have time, the gym is too expensive, I don't know how to do it. Excuses are easy. I've got a million of 'em. But if you want to get fit or lose weight then you must stop making excuses. At least tell the truth to yourself, if no one else.

If you watch a crappy soap opera every day you have time to exercise. If you hit the snooze button half a dozen times before getting out of bed in the morning, you have time to exercise. If you can't afford a gym, you can do it at home to a DVD, or simply run outside. All you need is a pair of trainers.

If you really want to do it badly enough then you will find the way. Many people don't want to enough. This is why there are always more people down the pub, than in the gym.

Parkrun

As I said a little earlier, exercising with others is one way to make it a little more fun as well as motivate you along the way too.

If you are thinking about giving running a try then parkrun is a great place to start. They take place in many parks across the country (and all over the world), always at 9am on a Saturday and always a 5K. Any ability is welcome to take part. It is timed and to join in you just have to register on their website in advance of taking part. Best of all, it is entirely free.

My local parkrun is in Leeds. It is a double 2.5K loop with a big hill in the middle. It is a truly horrible hill. I am very much a fair weather runner so only turn up in the summer, but it is 52-week of the year thing if you don't mind running in the rain.

At one my first parkruns, I got to the end of the first loop and all the volunteers cheered and shouted encouragement. I waved at them, thinking how nice and supportive they were. And then realised that just behind me was a man finishing the whole thing is about 18 minutes. Oh well.

One of the best things about parkrun is that it is both competitive and not at all competitive. There are those that turn up and run hard, striving for a PB. Often there are visiting running clubs with those that run regularly and competitively. But there are also folks that just walk the route with a dog or a pushchair just for the pleasure of it. Where there is a local café there's often a post run coffee or cake (or both).

The courses are marshalled, so you know where you are going. If you want to aim for a time there is often a pacer, wearing a helpful high-viz vest with the number of minutes they will cover the course in so that you can tag along behind them.

The volunteers are very welcoming and there are usually plenty of shouts of encouragement as you run around the course. When you cross the finish line you grab a token, take it to the marshal along with the barcode you get on registering, and you get emailed your time once the two are put together. Simple and lots of fun.

You can find your local parkrun by just going on their website: www.parkrun.org.uk. Give it a go – you might just like it!

Stuff I have learned from running

You get what you train for. Conversely, you don't get what you don't train for. You can't just turn up on the day and hope for the best.

Running slowly is still running.

By standing on the starting line of a race you are doing more than most people ever will.

When you are standing on that starting line, you have no idea what made you do this and you want to go home. This feeling will persist until you run over the finish line, when you realise it was awesome and want to sign up for another.

It is all about striving to beat your Personal Best, always.

You can only ever run your own race. Your only real competitor is yourself. It is just you versus the numbers.

Nothing tastes better than a Jelly Baby mid-way through a run.

The sound of your feet on the pavement is life.

When it comes to running you can't overthink it. You just have to put your trainers on and *go.*

Helping Hands

Sometimes in life you meet people that really help you along your journey and they don't even know it. At my first ever run with the Sweatshop beginners group run I was at the back. Obvs. Right at the *very* back. Just a 3K run, I half walked and half ran round the course.

I fell into running alongside one of the regulars who runs with the beginners group each week, timing the walking and running intervals and increasing them week on week to slowly build you up to running 5K. She ran with me all the way, encouraging me as I went. When we were in sight of the end of the run, she pushed me to run the final section as fast I could. This particular run finishes outside a large leisure complex where there's always plenty of people around outside. She told me to always come in running and to finish with a flourish. Advice that I have followed ever since.

At the end I puffed my thanks and off she went.

Not so long ago, I bumped into this girl at another exercise class and had the opportunity to say thank you to her. Thank you for running with me that very first time and keeping me going all the way around. Unsurprisingly she didn't remember me at all. I'm probably one of dozens of sweaty, gasping beginners she has nudged around those same streets. But I will remember her as being one of the first people to encourage me, when I didn't even believe in myself.

The next such person was my personal trainer. When I began to have the notion that I would do my first 10K, that just maybe this former fat girl could ran that far, I knew I would need some help.

My first PT session was about goals. Apparently, having a body that you would be happy to show any member of One Direction wasn't an appropriate goal. Who knew? So we agreed on running that 10K all the way. Slow would be acceptable, walking would not be. And as you know, I managed it.

My trainer has challenged, me, pushed me, guided me and listened to none of my bullshit. He has taught me that I have no limits. There has never been any question in his mind that I could achieve the events that I signed up for, so I didn't doubt it either.

There have been other helpers along the way too, especially at big events.

Sometimes when you are running a race, what makes it a little easier to keep on going when you think you can't run another step are those people that you meet so briefly; the kindness of strangers to just another runner passing by. Volunteers pointing the way and handing out the water, tidying up behind us, shouting encouragement over and over again to whoever runs on by.

Those people that held out Jelly Babies and Fruit Pastilles so that we could top up our energy levels. Children who hold out their hands for a high five all along the route. People who come out of their homes, sit in deckchairs or lean over their fences, shouting and cheering and waving flags. Those who hold signs, both funny and inspirational. Bands that play. Those that bother to check your name on your shirt and shout for you personally. Police officers on the route who join in with the encouragement. Every 'you are nearly there' even when you are not.

Your own family and friends, who hold your bags and wait patiently at the finish line to cheer you home.

Thank you, every one of you.

Thoughts on Personal Training

First things first. You don't have to have a Personal Trainer. Not everyone could afford one or wants that sort of commitment. If this isn't a route for you then you will find plenty of freely available exercise programmes that you can follow by yourself via You Tube and the like. Pinterest is another great place to find short exercise videos and guidance.

Having a Personal Trainer was however the differentiating factor for me. It took me from playing around with the idea of fitness to getting really serious about it.

So if it is something that interests you, here are my thoughts on what a Personal Trainer can do for you, and what you might want to think about when finding one.

First of all, the benefits.

Someone else is probably going to push you harder than you will ever push yourself. Even if you are the self-motivated type, a PT will make you do one more rep or lift a little more weight than you usually might.

They will get you to your goals faster. I have improved more in the last year more than I had in the previous three years combined.

They will challenge your bullshit excuses. I recently tried to tell my PT I didn't know why I had put weight on. His response? *"Yes. You really do."*

Their specialist knowledge. I've been a member of a gym for years. Including years in which I paid the monthly membership fee but never actually did anything apart from sitting in the Jacuzzi. But I had no idea that some of the stuff I was doing was at best sub-optimal, and at worse completely ineffectual.

If your motivation does decrease, the very fact that you are have an appointment to see someone and are paying for it will help to get you out of bed or off the sofa and into your gym gear.

You will not want to wimp out in front of your trainer and this will push you even further.

If you do decide to go ahead with personal training, here are a couple of recommendations from me.

Firstly, find someone you can build a good rapport with. And ideally swear in front of. Or at. I once told my PT I was going to buy a doll that looked like him and stick pins in it. You need to be able to be entirely honest about how you feel with your trainer. Fitness is as much a mental process as a physical one and that level of discussion needs to be present between you. If the rapport isn't there then change your trainer.

Be completely honest with your trainer. They will know if you are not, as the numbers don't lie. But if you aren't truthful about what are doing, eating, thinking and feeling, then they can't help you effectively.

According to an article I read recently, the personal training industry is about to get the Uber treatment. Put your requirements and location into an App and a PT will turn up within the hour. I can see why this might fit into the lifestyle of some busy folk. But for me this misses out on building the kind of relationship in which you can freely discuss goals, barriers and what success looks like. The process of discussion and refining your goals is helpful in its own right.

Do what they tell you to do. The chances are they know better than you do, unless you are similarly qualified. Even when I really dislike what my trainer tells me to do, I do it. Sometimes I moan about it but I do it all the same. Because that's the point. If it's about what I'd like to do, I'll go back in the Jacuzzi.

A few final points that might help you survive your sessions if you do get a personal trainer:

1. <u>Never</u> talk to them too much whilst you are doing cardiovascular exercise. They will take this as a sign that you are not exercising hard enough and will increase the torture level considerably.

2. Whilst lifting weights it is advisable to pull a few faces. Consider also including some 'I am in pain' grunting type noises towards the end of the set. Otherwise they will take this as a sign that the weight should increase significantly.

3. When they ask you how you are feeling about the intensity of the exercise on a scale of 1-10, never <u>ever</u> say less than 8. Otherwise they will take this as a sign you are not working hard enough and increase the torture level accordingly.

4. If you have an injury or health problem you should always tell your PT. However, <u>never</u> complain about being sore from a previous workout or tell them that you are tired. This is a signal to a PT that you are being a big lazy wuss and need to be appropriately dealt with.

5. Be aware that all Personal Trainers have a special watch. It measures a minute much more slowly than any other watch in the history of the world ever.

More Advice

So far you've had the pleasure of my collected thoughts on how to lose weight and how to get yourself exercising. You might be getting bored of me by now.

But if you're still along for the journey I'm now going to draw a little on my other life, as a Human Resources Director and Coach. Now I know that some people's experience with HR has been visiting their office for a disciplinary or meeting a very nice lady with a cardigan and a clipboard who made you sign a policy that you can't remember reading. I don't do that sort of HR. I do the sort of HR that is about how people behave, learn, think effectively and change. And this is what the next few chapters are all about.

First things first. Start with *WHY*.

Personal Trainers are encouraged to focus their clients on goals. It is all about what do you want to achieve and by when. Breaking it down into the small, medium and long term. Chunking it up into small parts to make it manageable. Keeping those goals under review and updating them. Weight loss classes do something similar by setting an initial weight loss target and monitoring against it each week.

That is the standard process and there is nothing wrong with it.

But it is missing something all the same.

It is missing why.

Because the why is the emotion. It is who you are and what you believe and how you got here. It is why you want this. It is your purpose and your focus. It is the thing that you come back to when it gets tough. When you think you can't, when the temptations come, it is your why that sees you through.

It is suggested by writers more qualified than me that, organisationally at least, where there is a strong 'why', a strong understanding of and association with purpose, then success is more likely. I think that applies to a weight loss journey too.

I had lots of answers to the why question.

- I wanted to wear nice, fashionable clothes from normal high street shops.
- I didn't want to feel sweaty and out of breath all the time.
- I no longer wanted to be embarrassed about what I looked like.
- I no longer wanted to feel so physically uncomfortable all the time.
- I was fed up.
- I wanted a nice photograph of me. Just one.
- I didn't want to go out again for a nice evening whilst looking like a sofa.

Of course, there is more than one "why" question that needs thinking about - a more difficult one to face perhaps. *Why did you put the weight on in the first place?*

In my experience there is often no one answer to this question. In coaching there is a saying; *the presenting issue is not the real issue.* This simply means that what might first appear to be the problem or the cause is anything but. There is surface stuff and then there is stuff buried further beneath. Dig deeper and the real issue is revealed.

We may never truly understand the reason why. It might just be too difficult to face. But as uncomfortable as it may be, it is a question worth reflecting upon all the same.

Why do you want to make this change? Why now? Why here? Who do you want to be tomorrow?

What has bought you to this place?

Start here.

Remember your why, always.

Goals. Keeping your eyes on the prize.

You've got to have a dream. Or how can you have a dream come true?

So goes the song anyway. Dreams are good. But goals are better. Ideally big, fat, hairy goals that scare you a little.

Goals are really important. Even more than you would think. One of my big early mistakes was not to have effective and well thought-through goals. During my diet years this was a big part of my problem. When I started those diets I was never specific about the goals. Because of my day job I know all about the importance of setting goals. At work, I know all about the evidence that says how those with detailed and documented goals are much more likely to achieve them. And yet I wasn't doing this for my own life. 'Losing weight' is not a goal. Neither is 'getting fit'. Much, much more specificity is needed.

One of the problems with these sorts of woolly and fuzzy aims is that they are just too big. That's one of the reasons why when you go to some weight-loss classes they talk to you about losing 10% of your body weight. This feels cognitively doable to most people when you turn that into pounds or kilos. Setting off on a journey to run a marathon when you can't currently run for a bus is daunting. Aiming to run a 5K significantly less so.

There is plenty of evidence to show that people who set formal goals, document them and keep them under review are more likely to achieve them. 'Losing weight' or 'getting fit' isn't a goal, it's a wish list. You need to articulate what you want and what success looks like. This will make it easier to focus and to achieve.

The official advice is that goals should be SMART: Specific, Measurable, Achievable, Realistic, Timed. This isn't a bad place to start even if it does lack a little emotion.

When I finally got around to setting some decent goals I found them hugely helpful.

During all of the diet years and the sofa years and the pretending to go the gym years, there was a black dress. I have worn it only once, to the wedding of a university friend a year or so after graduation. I wore it in that oh so brief moment in between losing a little of the university weight and then beginning the slippery slope towards obesity. My Dad bought me the dress. It was from House of Fraser and it cost £100, a little bit glamorous for someone paying back a student loan. A black wrap-around, knee length dress that made me look like I had a waist. In all of the years that I was too fat for the dress, when every other item of clothing went by the way of the charity shop, I never threw away the dress. I remembered how I felt when I wore it and I knew that one day I wanted to feel like that again. I had a clear vision in my mind of how I would look and how I would feel. And there is another lesson right there.

Having a vision to hold onto is key to getting you through a difficult day when you feel like throwing in the towel and eating all of the things. Another thing that I have learned from my day job is the importance of writing that vision down and bringing it to life and regularly coming back to it. I recommend giving it a go. If you write your own personal vision, then make it real, make it colourful, and make it aspirational.

When the weight finally began to come off, I would hold the dress against me to see how close I was getting to wearing it again. Then I got to the stage where I could get it over my head, even if I couldn't zip it up.

And then... it fitted.

I planned to wear it to an event. After more than 12 years, I would wear that dress again. Only when it actually came to the day of the event it was too big. The dress still hangs in my wardrobe. A dress that might only have been worn once but had represented all hopes and dreams.

When I started working with my personal trainer we put together more formal goals. I had a specific weight target, and the aim to run that 10K, all the way.

Think about your goals.   Write them down.   Review them often.
Recognise your progress. Smash those goals and then set new ones.

What does your new life look like?

Habits and Triggers

There is much written about habits - how you make them and how to break them.

It is sometimes said that you are what you repeatedly do.

It is also said that if you do what you have always done you will get what you have always got.

When it comes to weight loss and fitness, there are elements of truth in both.

So much of what we do is habit. Up to 70%, or so I have read. A lot of what we think are conscious decisions are anything but. We are simply going through our days, following our usual habits and responding to the same old triggers.

It seems like the science still can't quite get to the bottom of how long it takes to both form a new habit or to get rid of an old one. What is clear is that when we are trying to build new habits, repetition is key. That's why you will find plenty of fitness apps, all built around doing something every day, such as the 30-day Abs challenge and the like.

When we do something for the first time it is often difficult, simply because it is new. We have no knowledge to fall back on, no experience. But when we do that new thing, the action builds a whole neural new pathway in our brain. When we repeat the activity, that neural pathway gets bigger and stronger and so it gets easier. We remember and reinforce. A habit is born.

Think about learning to throw and catch a ball as a child. The first time we may fumble and drop that ball. With repetition our skill develops. We get better and better at handling the ball until the action becomes second nature – an unconscious action to reach and catch (unless you are me of course).

We need habits and routines. They make our lives easier. We don't want to have to get up in the morning and have to figure out all over again how to get dressed and get to work. We don't need to have to plan how to clean our teeth. We have a routine and we just ease into it – pre-programmed habit loops. Unfortunately however, these automatic brain processes that are designed to help us can also work against us too, especially when we are trying to make changes in our lives.

Have you ever smoked? I did, for years. If you have too then I bet just like me your smoking took place at very similar times or following very similar triggers. One when you first arrive at work. A second, about mid-morning. Always one after a meal. Always one with a drink in the pub. And so on.

Eating is often habitual. Triggered by something in particular. The same old same old. Long laid down. Big fat neural pathways ready for us to slip into.

A takeaway on a Saturday night.

The Sunday roast.

Something sweet after a meal.

A little snack about 3pm in the office.

A fry-up because it is the weekend.

A bad day at work equals a glass of wine to cheer you up.

A certain time of day that you normally eat a meal.

A social event.

An argument with a friend that leads you to reach for the biscuit tin.

Losing weight and getting fit is about breaking old habits and making newer, healthier ones. It is about understanding and recognising your triggers so that you control them rather than allowing them to control you.

About habits and triggers I have some good news and I have some bad news. The good news is that you don't have to be controlled by your own habits. Bad habits can be broken and new and better ones can be formed. The bad news is that it takes conscious, sustained effort. Even when you think you have cracked a habit, your brain will sometimes have a last ditch attempt at pulling you back, often in periods of difficulty or stress. The bad habits are always there, sleeping. We just have to learn how to manage them. Replace bad habits with good.

The first step to beating your habits and triggers is understanding them and recognising them when they arise. Then you have the opportunity to avoid your old pre-programmed habit loops and doing what you have always done. A food diary is a standard recommendation that I've also made in this little book. Another diary worth keeping for a few weeks is one that records when you eat. When do the cravings arise? What prompts you to head for the fridge? What makes you want to cheat a little or give into temptation?

Maybe it's one of those things listed above. Maybe it is the EastEnders theme tune because that's when you normally sit down and have a biscuit and a cuppa. Maybe it is when you have an argument with your other half. Finishing the kids' leftovers automatically. Maybe it is just because it is the weekend. Maybe it is an emotion.

Bring conscious thought to your eating habits. Make a note of how you feel before you eat. Recognise what you are doing automatically, without conscious thought. Then try a few of these practical ideas about creating new habits.

- Set reminders on your phone or use this facility on a wearable if you have one. Set it to prompt you to drink water several times a day at the same time or to get up and walk around.
- Only tackle a couple of habits at a time otherwise your willpower will get depleted. Give it a few weeks before tackling others. You may even decide to just go with one change to begin with and that's just fine. Believe it or not, willpower works very much like a muscle. It can get stronger through use but it can get tired too from overuse.
- Prepare your food in advance. I know that this is time consuming. But if you make your lunch the night before work,

you will take it and you will eat it. If you don't you might just end up scoffing from the vending machine.

- Reward yourself: just do it differently. Food is nice. Wine is nice. Meals out with friends are nice. They provide us with a reward, from the taste itself to the experience through to what it accompanies. So reward yourself with something else. Buy yourself a treat at the end of the week if you have stuck to your goals.
- Look at your habits and triggers diary and take action accordingly. If it's a chocolate bar mid- afternoon that's your habit then make sure you have something better to eat instead ready and waiting on your desk.
- Replace the habit. If you love a big glass of orange juice then swap it for orange squash. If you just have to have a coffee on the way to work then go for the Skinny version not the one with the caramel shot. Swap the Friday night takeaway curry for one you have made yourself. Replace bad with better.
- Exercise at the same times. Morning is best if you can, before your brain can figure out what you are up to. Make it easy for yourself by getting everything ready the night before. Get up and just JFDI. It will soon feel become a routine and the horror of the early rise will wear off – I promise!
- Monitor your progress. Try apps and wearables or a good old fashioned pedometer if you have one to track your steps. Take note of what you are achieving.
- Reflect on what you have done well. Progress is progress even it is only a small step. Next time take a slightly bigger one.
- Make it easy to be successful. So whatever food is your go to temptation, clear it out of the house. Build momentum slowly. Trust that the results will come.
- Make a list. Write down the habits you want to break and the new ones you want to make. Then tick them off as you go.

You've got this.

Stuff that stops you

There is plenty that will get in the way when it comes to both weight loss and fitness alike. There are barriers both real and imagined that can derail our attempts to make changes in our lives.

But ultimately, I believe that the biggest barrier with any weight loss of fitness programme is simply, yourself.

Research has been undertaken by the fitness industry about why people start exercise regimes but don't follow them through. The standard advice for the general population is to do a minimum of 30 minutes of cardiovascular exercise at least three times a week. Only the research found that for many people that was just too much of a change to cope with and sustain.

Work, childcare, finances, family, housework, lifestuff. There is plenty to stop us finding the time to work out, to go for that run, to prepare healthy food or get to that weight loss group. These are usually presented as extrinsic barriers – in other words, outside of the control of the individual. If these really are the reasons of course. Because sometimes these are just convenient excuses. Sometimes it is really about motivation. And few of us face up the fact that sometimes the real reason is that we don't exercise or sort our diet out is that we simply can't be bothered.

All change starts with motivation to do so. The desire for something different. We are back to that moment again – the push that makes you take action. Without motivation and a deep desire for change then the barriers can seem unsurmountable. When the motivation kicks in, when the tipping point is reached, that list of problems look like nothing more than mild inconveniences.

And then there is self-sabotage. Self-sabotage is a real problem with many overweight people. It may sounds like a strange turn of phrase, even a difficult concept to get your head around. That we might want something so very badly and yet deliberately get in our own way. But if you've ever started a diet and then cut yourself a slice of cake, skipped a gym class because it's raining, or ordered a takeaway not too long afterwards, then this is exactly what you are engaged in.

There are other ways that we stop ourselves.

Take these.

I have worked really hard all week, so I deserve a treat.

It's Saturday night, so it's takeaway night.

It's my birthday / Christmas / Easter / holidays / Valentine's Day etc. so I'll just eat that cake / mince pie / chocolate, and so on.

If you say any of these things then you are falling victim to what I call the Special Treat Fallacy. A way of pretending to yourself that it's okay to cheat. You are trading what you want now for what you want most. You are making excuses to yourself.

There are techniques that Personal Trainers learn to get people motivated and keep them there. Most courses teach the stages of behavioural change. Models and stages.

I'm not sure I believe it is entirely possible to motivate someone else to change their lives. You need to find your own reasons, no-one can do it for you. All the nagging in the world won't get you very far. That theory of behavioural change often talks about the stages that people go through. One of them is called 'pre-contemplation'. Which basically means thinking about something but not doing it. Buying some trainers but never putting them on. Joining a gym but never turning up. Buying lots of healthy food and then throwing it away at the end of the week when it's gone past its best. I was stuck in the pre-contemplation stage for years. I thought long and hard about exercise, from the Jacuzzi in my gym.

Here's the thing. There is plenty that will get in the way of you achieving your goals, if you let it. Stuff that gets in the way is a decision. A choice. You either let it or you don't. It is that simple.

If the only thing stopping you reaching your goal weight or achieving your fitness goals is you, why *are* you getting in your own way?

Plateau

Sometimes you hit a plateau; you are trying hard to lose weight and doing all of the right things, but the rate of loss slows down or stops all together.

It has happened to me several times during the last few years and it isn't at all unusual.

There are a few reasons why this might happen. The first is simple; your body is adjusting to a new regime. It will get used to fewer calories and more exercise. So when a plateau occurs sometimes it is simply about keeping on going; trust the process and the results will eventually come. Occasionally you might need to up your game a little. Time to tackle another habit, time to add in a little more exercise.

Of course, it might also be habit creep. A few of those old bad food habits sneaking back in. A few extra calories here or there, perhaps a skipped workout, all adding up to a standstill on the scales.

But never lose sight of the fact that slow progress is still progress. Hang on in there.

Just one important thing. Make sure that it's really a plateau. And it isn't our old friend Denial paying another visit.

Here's a story from me just to illustrate the point.

A few months ago I engaged in some high level whining to my Personal Trainer.

I was complaining about how long my weight had been unchanged. How I was stuck. How six months of slogging away in the gym had delivered me not the loss of one single pound. And about how this was completely and utterly unfair.

And then he asked me one question.

What have you actually changed in that last six months?

I bluffed it out. Defended myself. Argued that I had, at great personal sacrifice, entirely given up wine.

He pointed out to me that I had given up alcohol two weeks ago and that it therefore didn't count, yet at least.

And then he asked me again.

What have you actually changed during that six months you are complaining about?

Leaving me to concede……. Nothing.

I hadn't made any changes so I could not in turn expect any miracles. The same calories consumed, the same level of effort in the gym. I hadn't put in the additional effort, so the reward wasn't on its way.

You've probably heard this quote: 'Do what you have always done and get what you have always got'.

Case in point.

Questions to ask yourself

As I've said already, my day job is in Human Resources. As part of that role I coach leaders in our business. Coaching is basically about getting people to think for themselves. So often in life we are surrounded by people who want to give us advice and tell us what they think. If you are trying to lose weight you will meet a lot of these people. Coaching is different. It is about asking people a question and then allowing them to have the space to work something out for themselves.

When you are training to be a coach there is a model that is often taught, and it is a helpful and simple structure for fitness and weight loss too. It is just a way of thinking about your current challenge and how you will tackle it.

It goes like this.

Goal, Reality, Options, Will.

GROW.

We've talked about goals. It is what you are trying to achieve. Goals can be big and hairy and ever so slightly scary, or they can equally be about taking small steps. There is power in both, so do what works for you is my only advice.

Reality is about the now. It is about looking in the mirror – metaphorically and quite possibly actually. What is your current situation? How does that compare with the goal, and where you want to be? How big is the gap? What is going on for you right now that is relevant to what you want to achieve?

Options are simple. What are you able to do about it? What options do you have, and which ones do you want to take?

And finally, Will. In other words, will you actually do it? If you have made the promises before, started the diets and begun the exercise regime, this time, will you keep it up?

There are some coaching questions that I use all the time when I am working with leaders. There are the ones that I find most useful to get people thinking. I've put some of them here as I believe that they apply to weight loss and fitness too. Maybe grab yourself a pen, take a few moments to reflect, and write down your answers.

What is holding you back?

What is going to get in the way of your goal? How will you overcome that?

On a scale of 1-10, how committed are you to making this change? And if it is less than five, why are you even reading this book?

What are the three actions you could take straight away that help you towards your goal?

If you knew you could achieve all of your goals, what would you do?

What is the excuse that you always use?

What would you do if you weren't scared?

When I said I was writing this little book, a friend suggested that some readers might be interested in knowing what my routine and diet was for maintaining the weight loss

So here goes.

I aim to train nearly every day for an hour. Most of the time I make this work and frankly sometimes I don't, depending on work, family and all that other life stuff. Usually training for me is early in the morning before work because that is just when I can fit it in.

So it is carbs for breakfast to give me the energy to work out. Many trainers will recommend eggs for breakfast. It is very good advice. I just have neither the time nor inclination to make them at 6am, so I stick with granary toast. If you can find the desire put a poached egg on top.

My exercise is a real mixed bag. Over the course of the week I will do a few sessions of cardio, combined with some swimming, weight training and a mix of classes – usually HIIT and Pilates. I should run but often I don't. If the sun is out then so might my bike be. I don't usually have a rest day. This is also not advisable. Rest is part of the programme and is when progression takes place. Another case of do as I say, not as I do......

I snack mid-morning. Something with protein in it that will satisfy the hunger pangs and get me through until lunch. Often, this is some natural Greek yoghurt with a banana or berries, or a handful of nuts and seeds. Dreadfully boring I know. Sorry about that.

Lunch is usually a salad, always with some sort of protein. Eggs, fish, chicken or turkey. Homemade until the end of the week when there is nothing left in the fridge. Then it is straight to M&S to see what they have on the shelves. It is possible to get healthy food of the shop-bought variety, you just have to be careful to read the nutritional labels and check the calorie, fat and sugar content. If you often eat on the go then watch out for food and drink that is usually loaded with sneaky extra calories, like speciality coffees, smoothies and pre-packed sandwiches.

Mid-afternoon, another snack. Often a protein bar if I am out and about just for ease. Otherwise it might be some slow release carbs.

As for the evening, I'd like to say that I eat only protein and vegetables. Lean, home prepared foods. That would be a lie. Several nights a week I am good. I will prepare my own soups or pasta sauces (easier than you think, cheaper than the supermarket, and distinctly lower on additives, sugar, salt and other nasties). Most of the time it will be chicken, eggs, turkey and the like. It will be a healthy recipe from a lean cookbook. Only if I am to be entirely truthful, some evenings when I am busy it is beans on toast. Other nights, just every so often, I might throw caution to the wind and order a takeaway. If I didn't I probably would have lost those extra pounds, hit my target weight or be more often squeezing into that elusive size eight.

Oh well.

As for other food, the truth is I often don't eat what I'd like to. When the doughnuts come round in the office I would like one. When the work canteen serves sausage and mash I'd very much love a big plateful ideally with a side portion of chips. Sometimes, I go out for a meal with friends and don't have a drink. I'd like one of course, but in reality it doesn't make the evening worse not to have one.

In my bigger days, I had a bit of a problem with bread. Croissants and iced buns and French bread covered in butter and brie. Soft white rolls filled with bacon and sausage. Toast with lashings of butter and marmalade. Chip butties. Garlic bread with everything. Bread sticks dipped in humus. Bread on the side. Bread as the meal. Bread, bread, bread. I ate it with nearly every meal. So that had to be rationed too. Now, if I eat bread it is only of the dark, rye type, and never more than once a day.

I choose not to drink much. I hate to break it to you but a large glass of wine is basically a doughnut in a glass. Sugar and empty calories with no nutritional value at all. I don't drink much coffee and I go to bed no later than 10pm every night. Sleep is part of the programme.

And yes, you are right. This is really very boring.

I also chose not to eat white pasta and rice, creamy sauces or too much shop-bought stuff. I religiously read the back of packets for nutritional labels so that I understand what I am eating.

On weekends I ease up a bit. That approach does slow down the achievement of your goals but frankly there are only so many chicken breasts a girl can eat before she needs a pizza.

I drink a lot of water (a minimum of two litres a day) and as a result spend a lot of time in the toilet.

Much of this advice you will probably have heard before. There's nothing new here. I'm sorry about that too.

Sticking to these decisions is simply down to discipline. Thinking about what you want most rather than what you want now. The problem is we are very, very bad at balancing what we want now as opposed to what we want longer term. As for me, sometimes now wins out, and sometimes it doesn't. Just one of those things I am still working on.

And finally.....

If I have made it look like I've got it all sorted, that I am a success, then it's time to me to come clean. I haven't. I probably never will. My journey is ongoing, and probably always will be.

As I write this particular chapter, I am just three pounds away from my target weight. But this weekend I went seriously off the rails. A family trip to Centre Parcs. Over the three days I have consumed: a large iced donut, a Crunchie, two tubs of pick and mix, a large bag of popcorn, a family sized bag of Doritos, three fairy cakes with buttercream icing, a bag of giant chocolate buttons and created a local Prosecco shortage.

Because once the 'after' pictures have been published, after the cameras on the weight loss TV show have stopped rolling, after the "well done you" congratulations and the new clothes and target weight has been reached......

Then what?

I'm going to hazard a guess. For most people the struggle continues. Always.

Many diets fail. The percentages about how many people put all the weight back on and then some, are huge (no pun intended).

Why?

For some of the reasons I have already talked about in this little book.

Because we try and make too big a change all at once.

Because we see diets as a discrete event rather than a way of eating and living.

Because we do fad diets that aren't sustainable over the long term.

Because food is lovely. Especially cake.

Because we don't address the real reasons that we got fat in the first place.

Because our bad habits are ingrained and sometimes pull us back.

Because it is hard.

I have accepted that I will always, always struggle with food. I will always want to eat the things that I shouldn't, eat more than I need to, crave all of the bad stuff. I will always from time to time fall right off the wagon.

It is what it is.

When it comes to fitness and to weight loss, there are still two sides to me. I wear two faces. And in my every day it goes a little bit like this;

I don't want to get up at this time in the morning and go to training. Why on earth am I doing this? I have had ENOUGH.

Oooohh, I'm in the gym and I feel AWESOME.

I really hate running.

I feel like going for a run.

(At a running event, standing on the start line). Why am I here? WHY? I hate running.

(Afterwards). Yeay that was awesome!!!

I definitely don't need any new gym clothes. I have a lot of gym clothes.

Look at those fabulous leggings. Buy all the things!

I am strong. I have willpower.

CAKE.

It doesn't matter what I weigh. This is not the most important measure of my success.

I have put a pound on!!!!! WTAF?

I can't lift that.

Oh yes I can!

I can Zumba like a boss.

looks in mirror I have no co-ordination whatsoever. I look like a frolicking hippopotamus.

Protein, protein, protein.

CAKE.

I totally need a rest day. They are really important to let your muscles recover. Today will be a rest day.

I can't stop thinking about going to the gym.

I feel great when I eat good, clean food. I feel rubbish when I eat junk. So I will do the former.

CAKE.

And so on.

Very Final Thoughts.

There is much I have learnt along my journey during the last three and a half years or so. The first is that this is your journey and yours alone. Others may stand by your side or cheerlead you on. Others won't believe you can do this and some might even laugh at you.

But this is your journey and only you can take the steps.

Today, I am so far from where I once was. But my journey is most definitely not finished. Because there is no finishing line.

I don't have a magazine perfect body. I have accepted that I will never have one. Not unless you can get airbrushing in real life. I still want to eat all of the food in the 'before' sections of the magazines. There are still days when I give into temptation.

I am in fact, a work in progress. Something that I am just fine with. I will continue to improve myself every day.

I lost weight, and I gained a new life.

My most important learning is simply this; weight loss begins in the mind. It is not only about what you eat but what you believe. As the saying goes, if you think you can, you can. If you think you can't, then you can't. This sounds simple. Like a throwaway line. Maybe it is, but in clichés there is also truth.

If you are reading this book, maybe you are on a journey. Maybe you are thinking about beginning one. Wherever you are on your path I wish you every success. Believe in yourself. Be stronger than your excuses.

If this girl can do it, you can do it.

Do it for the health of it. Do it to make yourself proud.

You've got this.

Postscript

Today I ran a half marathon.

As I've said before, I don't really like running. I'm not entirely sure why I signed up for it, apart from the fact that it seemed like another achievement to tick off the list. Another item of proof in the list of things that demonstrate I am now someone else.

The general dislike of all things running had spilled over into the training. Give me a choice of exercise and I'll pick the gym every time. So as a result I hadn't done nearly as much I should have done.

I knew it was going to be hard.

I knew that aiming for a time wasn't going to be an option.

I had just one goal: get round the whole course. Get round it by running all the way and try not to die whilst doing it.

A week before the event the weather was forecast to be rain. But the day dawned sunny and warm. Too warm. I rocked the tomato look all the way around.

If you have never taken part in a large event, I encourage you to sign up for something. Anything. Even if you think you can't do it. Because most of the time those things that we think we can't do, we really can.

Standing on the starting line of an event is an amazing feeling. The noise, the colour, the nerves, the anticipation. At a running event I am always taken at the start, when all the runners are bunched up together, by the noise of all those feet slapping on the pavement in some sort of strange rhythm. I'm taken too by the generosity of those that turn out and shout for you. That wave signs. Play instruments. That come out of their homes and cheer you on.

Today, the generosity of those folks including turning a garden hosepipe into an impromptu shower in which we could cool down. A house blaring out the theme tune to 'Chariots of Fire'. And the oh so lovely folks at about mile seven who had set up a stall outside their house with orange segments and Jelly Babies.

I was, to be entirely honest, less happy about being overtaken by a man some twenty years older than me who did the entire route skipping.

The first couple of miles, up and down hills. Some of them distinctly challenging. By mile five I found my stride, powering down an unknown dual carriageway somewhere on the outskirts of Leeds. But by mile ten my thighs had decided that it was time to stop all this silliness and have a nice sit down.

Running that last half a mile was both terrible and amazing. Terrible for the pain in my legs and hips. But made amazing by the noise of the crowd, the music, the cheering, the knowing it was nearly over, the sight of the finish line. Powering home that last two hundred yards.

My time was a fairly respectable 2 hours 30 minutes and 33 seconds. Damn those 33 seconds.

Next time I will be faster.

Now I'm typing these last few words whilst lying on the sofa, a celebratory glass of Prosecco within arm's reach.

My legs hurt.

My feet hurt.

I am knackered.

And I feel awesome.

After all this, there is one thing that I am now completely sure of.

I am never, ever doing a full marathon.

Probably.

Acknowledgements and further reading

As I've said somewhere else in this book, when I am not in the gym or trying not to eat Mint Matchmakers, I work in Human Resources and I am a qualified coach (the business kind, not the sport kind). As unusual as this might at first sound, I've found there to be real parallels between my day job and my fitness hobby.

Performance at work is also about goal setting, focus, feedback, prioritisation, planning and adapting the plan as you go along. Coaching in particular is about helping people be the best that they can be and making them resourceful.

Some of what has helped me over the last three or so years has been drawn not just from the world of fitness but from my professional role too. So if you are interested in any of the topics I have mentioned throughout this little book, here are a few of my recommendations for further reading:

If you want to know more about the importance of having a vision and the regular reinforcement of it, then read 'Day Dreams' by Simon Clarkson.

If you want to know more about habits and how our brain works with them, then read 'The Power of Habit' by Charles Duhigg.

If you want to know more about that stuff about starting with why, then read Simon Sinek, 'Start with Why'. Lots of application to work and to life.

If you want a simple introduction to coaching and the GROW model, try 'Don't Just Manage, Coach' by Ben Morton.

If you want to read more of my ramblings, you can follow my fitness blog http://allaboutfitness.org/

If you want some awesome design work, try Simon Heath who designed the cover to this book. He is on Twitter as @SimonHeath1

Printed in Great Britain
by Amazon

42462635R00061